power of the seed

A GUIDE TO OILS FOR HEALTH & BEAUTY

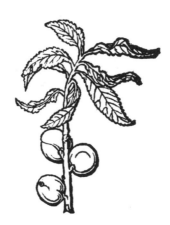

SUSAN M. PARKER

process self-reliance series

This publication contains the opinions and ideas of its author. It is intended to provide
helpful and informative material on the subjects addressed in the publication.

Power of the Seed is part of the Self-Reliance Series. For further information about these
titles, see: *www.processmediainc.com*

Process Media
1240 W. Sims Way Suite 124
Port Townsend, WA 98368

Copyedited by Bess Lovejoy
Cover design by Gregory Flores
Interior design by Lissi Erwin / Splendid Corp.

Many, but not all botanical illustrations are from *Herbarum Imagines Vivae*, Frankfurt,
Germany, 1535.

Technical and chemical diagrams by the author.

Typeset in Minister Std Book with Steagal, Goudy Bookletter 1911, Calvert Std
and Rockwell Italic.

ISBN 978-1934-17054-0
Printed in the United States of America
10 9 8 7 6 5 4

power
of
the
seed

Contents

Acknowledgements ix

Introduction to Oils 1

My Oil Story 4
Let's Look at the Lipids 9
Terms: What is Essential? 10

Chapter One: Oils of the Plant World 13

Lipids and the Fixed, Carrier, and Base Oils 14
Essential Oils 16
Spiritual Nature of Oils 19
Regional Differences in Oil-Bearing Plants 20
Oils in Human Culture 21

Chapter Two: Lipid Structure and Chemistry 101 22
The Structure of Fixed Oils

Fatty Acids and Triglycerides 23
The Carbon Chains 25
Fatty Acids 26
Saturated Oils and Fatty Acids 27
Unsaturated Fatty Acids 30
Monounsaturated Fatty Acids 32
Polyunsaturated Fatty Acids 32
Super/Polyunsaturated Fatty Acids 33
Unsaturated Fatty Acids and Oxygen 34
The Ends of the Carbon Chains 35
Naming Fatty Acids 36
Shorthand or Coded System of Fatty Acids 36
Fatty Acid Names 37
Omega Classification 39

Chapter Three: Beyond Fatty Acids ... 40

... to Oils 41
Comparing Two Oils: Olive and Cocoa Butter 43

Chapter Four: Whole Oils—Qualities, Values, Refining 45

Saponification Value 45
Unsaponifiable Portion 46
Iodine Value of Oils 47
Peroxide Value and Acid Value 47
Fractionation 48
Refining Oils 49

Chapter Five: Other Forms of Lipids 51

Phospholipids—Lecithin 51
Waxes 53
Trans Fats & Oils 53
Petrochemicals—Mineral Oil 56
Sperm Whale Oil 57

Chapter Six: Consuming Fatty Acids—Oils and Health 59

The Essential Nutrients 60
Essential Fatty Acids and Health 62
Important but Not "Essential" 64
Medium-Chain Fatty Acids 65

Chapter Seven: Topically—Oils and the Skin 67

The Skin Is an Organ 68
Fatty Acids, Sebum, and the Skin 70
Allergens, or Everyone Is Allergic to Something 71
Oils and Problems of Skin Health 72
Oils and Skin Aging 74
Oils, Sun, and Tanning 75
Oils and Skin Care 76

Chapter Eight: Common and Important Fatty Acids for the Skin 77

Essential and Polyunsaturated Fatty Acids 77

Monounsaturated Fatty Acids 79
Saturated Fatty Acids 81
Very-Long-Chain Fatty Acids 83
Unique and Uncommon Fatty Acids 85

Chapter Nine: Phyto-Chemicals 88

The Necessity of Oxygen and Antioxidants 89
Phenolic Compounds 90
Flavonoids 91
Non-Flavonoid Phenolic Acids 93
Hydroxycinnamates 94
Lignans 96
Terpenes and Terpenoids 96
Vitamins 98

Oils, Butters, and Waxes: A List 104

Abyssinian to Yangu 106

Natural Waxes Used in Skin Care 188

Working with Natural Oils 193

Care and Handling of Oils 193
Using Oils on the Skin 195
Facial Care with Natural Oils 196
Cleansing with Oils 196
Facial Oils or Serums 201
Oils for Massage 211
Simple Body Scrubs 213
Whipped Salves & Body Butters 215
Oils and Herbs 218
Infusing Herbs in Oil 218
Salve-Making 226

Appendices 235

Oils by Use 236
Oils by Properties 240
Oils by Source 248
Botanical Families of Oil-Bearing Plants 252

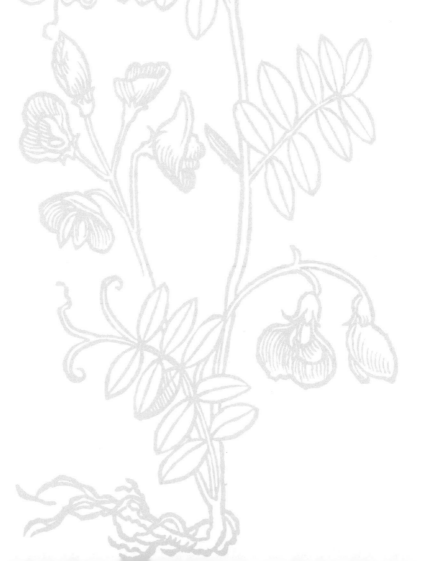

Saponification Values for 90 Oils, Fats, and Waxes 259
Fatty Acid Families of Oils 262
Listing of Common Fatty Acids by Saturation and Omega Family 264
Fatty Acid Tables and Composition for the Oils 268
Measurements & Equivalents 296
Essential Oil Dilutions by Percentage 297
Glossary of Terms 298

Bibliography 313

Sources 318

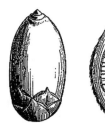

Acknowledgements

Books are seldom written or produced in a vacuum. People help, we pick up bits of information here and there, and knowledge accumulates. Then, when a book comes together, we want to thank all those who helped it come into being. This project has had a long period of incubation and several iterations over more than a dozen years. Some links and sources of information have faded into history. But others stand out as turning points in understanding.

Not being a chemist and only taking one class in college, understanding the structure and basic chemistry of the fatty acids and lipids in a meaningful way was a challenge. Information can be gleaned from books or websites but the basics, the fundamentals, are often hard to grasp without knowledgeable help. Two friends who are also chemists by training stepped into this space of ignorance to bring the clarity that only the trained mind can. Bob Lindberg of Santa Rosa, California, helped me grasp the basics of soap-making when I was beginning this journey. He helped with the explanation of how oil is transformed with the action of lye to form soap. That meant understanding what the oils were composed of in the first place, their structure and chemistry. His introduction was invaluable.

Fast-forward a dozen years and my good friend Lyn Faas of Port Townsend, Washington, helped with the phrasing and language to clarify the basic chemistry of the subject. A fundamental misunderstanding about the nature of fatty acids was gently corrected so that the true nature of the molecules was presented accurately. Lyn was generous with her time and knowledge, helping to fix and adjust language and concepts so that the material is accurate.

Books too played a part, and Udo Erasmus' *Fats That Heal, Fats That Kill* enabled me to take what I had learned from my work with Bob Lindberg and soap-making and fill in missing links and gaps in understanding. Erasmus' book presents the chemistry of oils and lipids in great depth, including both the natural and manipulated forms. Along with books, a wide variety of websites provided information on all aspects of the subject. From small and obscure sites to those from universities, government agencies, and research institutions, each answered the questions that came up along the way. Suppliers of oils too, have researched their materials and make this information available on the web. Natural Sourcing LLC., in particular, has much information and a wide variety of oils to offer. The process of writing this book has been one of self-education. I am indebted to each of the very many sources available to me.

I also want to thank Gail Julian, fellow herbalist, long-time supporter of my work and muse, for reigniting the flame under the earlier version of this project.

As you may or may not know, the first attempts at publishing this material was self-instigated. In those days it was still cut and paste, which made for a fun, if challenging, art project. But real publishing of real books has been an eye opener. I am deeply indebted to Process Media for seeing the value in this work and bringing it into being.

Thank you Juliet Parfrey for your introduction to your brother Adam Parfrey and to Adam for Process Media and its vision; Jessica Parfrey, for your guidance and all the back-end work bringing the book into being, including distribution and keeping me on track. Thank you Bess Lovejoy, for your excellent comments, suggestions, and smoothly flowing editing style that made the text readable and clear. Lissi Erwin for the beautiful book design and ability to organize illustrations, charts, technical data into clear readable form that enhances the material. Monica Rochester for helping track down many of the illustrations and images. And all the others that I don't know but that will bring this project into form, including printers, and distributors that have a hand in getting this into the world.

I have acknowledged others for helping with technical information, but any inaccuracies that may remain in the text or descriptions are mine alone. The lack of formal background in chemistry has had its pros and cons. The way I present the chemical structure and workings of the fatty acids, I am told, is unorthodox. Yet my curiosity kept me at the task of making connections and linking relevant information to the subject. The sum total of my inquiry is contained here and my need for a reference manual is complete. I share it with others who have need of information on the many and important fatty acids, lipids, and oils of the botanical world.

Acknowledgements are never complete until the author's support crew, their family, are recognized for the untold help they provide. I thank my husband Jeryl for reading reams of early drafts and acting as sounding board for the ideas and concepts as they bubbled up; his help is far beyond what I can ever fully acknowledge. And my daughter Olivia, who has taken to the oils with a passion dear to her mother. My son Evan, his wife Sarah, and grandbaby Theo, have proven willing guinea pigs trying out oil combinations for skin and body. And last but not least, the many friends and customers from around the country and world who have bought my products and provided invaluable feedback over the 18 or more years that this has been in production.

And finally, to my late mother, who I can still hear saying, "go look it up." She didn't believe that one needed to memorize information, just know where to find it. She also loved to read. When my form of dyslexia, a new concept then, revealed itself as I stumbled over the Dick, Jane, and Spot early readers, she took it upon herself to learn the new discipline of phonics. She spent hours and taught me how to break down and sound out words, to recognize them, and appreciate their ability to communicate. And so this book is dedicated to her and her exhortation "look it up," and the early intervention that helped me overcome my difficulty with reading. She opened up the world of the written word and made it accessible.

    —SMP

A Note on the Drawings

The fatty acid drawings represent the shapes and bonds between atoms in the fatty acid molecules, a visual representation of their basic structure. As molecules in nature, they are neither static nor absolute, while our drawings must be. The way the structures of the fatty acids change when nature, oxygenation, hydrogenation, and man act them upon is complex and dynamic, and difficult to represent in two-dimensional drawings, but we have done our best.

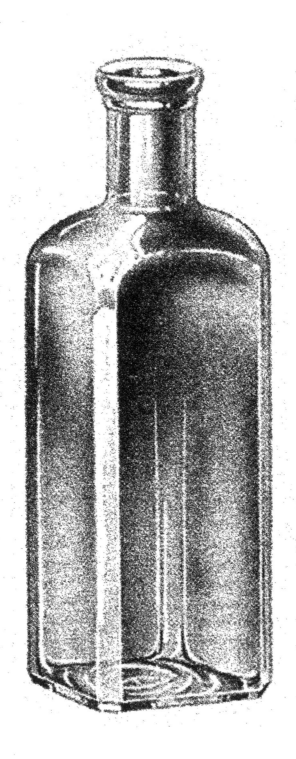

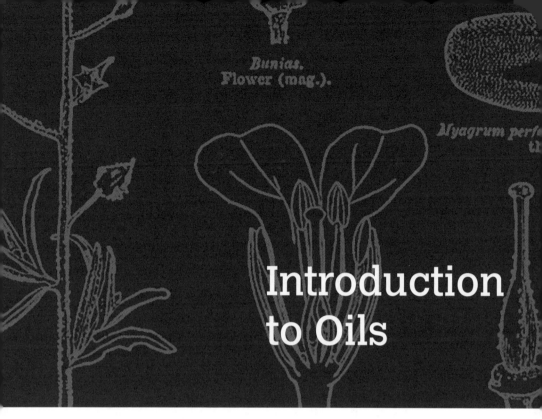

Introduction to Oils

Oils, beautiful, colorful, and vibrant, are nourishing, soothing, sensual, and medicinal. Occupying a place in nearly all aspects of life, from kitchen to spa, industry to clinic, oils are so much more than the pale-colored bottles on grocery shelves. There are countless oils representing all corners of the earth in every color, scent, taste, and texture, serving multiple purposes and functions. The world of plant-based oils is a large and fascinating place to study.Imagine people in far-flung parts of the world producing and using exotic oils. First, imagine central Africa, where the temperature is high and women are collecting fallen nuts, adding them to a large pot outdoors. The smoky scent of wood ash and oil heating fills the nose. The women are happy and talking while they work. At the end of the day, they will have oil for cooking, enough to oil the drum heads, and some oil left over to sell in the market. As they work, the oil separates from the nuts and rises to the surface of the pot. A few of the women pull a little of the oil off the surface and rub it into their skin to protect against the burning rays of the sun. Shea butter and oil are part of their daily activities, and their lives would not be the same without them.

In another corner of the world, imagine the olives are ripe this time of year. Days are spent collecting them to take to the pressing mill. The rich, spicy scent inside the mill house is a familiar and favorite smell. The oil will grace tonight's table in most of the dishes, and be shared with the rest of the family. Tomorrow is soap-making day for the oil that is not good enough for the kitchen and table. You could be in Italy, or Spain, or California in this scenario.

The world of plant oils is large and diverse. Culture by culture, around the globe and throughout time, oils are central players in all communities. Natural and necessary, the lubricant to nature's smooth functioning, oils are ever-present and integral to the life forms of plants, animals, and humans. The source for all this oil? **Seeds.** Seeds are nature's oil-producing calorie factories. A storehouse of sunshine within the seed, oils nourish the next generation of plant until it can feed itself through photosynthesis. Seeds and kernels, nuts, and fruiting bodies are complete energy and dietary centers, the grocers of the plant world.

Every seed has the capacity to make oil and carries unique properties from the parent plant. While all oils have a common structural similarity, each plant's seed brings something special to the individual commodity. Spicy, tangy olive oil is uniquely different from rich, flavorful, and solid coconut oil. Contrast similar oil dichotomies throughout the plant kingdom, and the range, variety, qualities, and properties possible become truly astonishing.

The goddess Flora, spirit of the plant world, produces an untold number of seeds each year. We eat some seeds all the time, such as sunflower and pumpkin. Others we toss, like watermelon seeds and olive pits. Often, seeds are undeveloped when we eat them and consumed unknowingly. But all seeds have the potential to produce oil when fully ripened. Under great pressure, gentle squeezing, or by chemical extraction, oils are separated from the rest of the seed matter.

Cultural, regional, communal, cooking, and healing traditions use local and native oils. Indigenous plants, those native to a particular geographical region, serve their communities by providing food and medicine locally. These oils are adapted to the specific climate and environmental conditions and to the local culture. By maintaining connections to native and indigenous flora, the community's continuity and health is preserved.

Rare and exotic or common and found closer to home, oils contain a variety of beneficial and useful properties for human endeavors. With modern means of distribution, we share oils from around the globe, enjoying their nourishing and culinary properties or using them in manufacturing and industrial applications. Sharing resources from communities other than our own, including native oils, unites us but also involves a level of responsibility. We must be conscious of the impact our desire for resources has on other places. Their culture, environment, and way of life deserve our respect and fair trade for their native goods.

Trees, wildflowers, grains, grasses, nuts, palms, shrubs, vegetables, and fruit, from every region, all produce seeds that can be and are pressed for oil. Globally, each region and type of plant produces a wide variety of oils. Color, scent, texture, nutritional compounds, and healing properties are broadly diverse. The many colors of oils range from red, orange, green, brown, golden yellows to completely clear. Each hue and tint carries attributes that give oils their own signature qualities, both nutritionally and for topical use.

In terms of scent, taste, texture, and feel, oils can be nutty or spicy, strongly green-smelling, fruity, thick and heavy, or light like water. Wide variations play a part in how oils are used and enjoyed. Who doesn't love a piece of French bread dipped in a good hearty olive oil, or coconut oil and its rich fatty milk in Indian food? The spicy oil of black cumin seed, nigella, is a delicacy of the Middle East and used medicinally there to heal the body.

Oil and fats have gotten a bad reputation in recent decades. Misunderstandings regarding their composition and how they function in the body, along with incomplete studies and the politics of the food industry, created a perfect storm of bad information and fear-based pronouncements. Oils are said to be bad for our health and to make us fat. Don't believe it! Fortunately, the information regarding oils and health is changing.

In fact, oils are vitally important to the healthy functioning of the body. Nutritionally, medicinally, and culinarily, oils are absolutely necessary for maintaining your physical body. Most importantly, however, oils are the food of the soul.

My Oil Story

The purpose of this book is somewhat self-serving. I wanted to create the reference manual I wished was available twelve years ago. The content will focus on oils for skin care, supported by nutritional, functional, and culinary information. We'll also take a few detours to look at common oils used in unusual ways, to demonstrate their functions as useful natural substances.

Plant oils can be of two kinds: the aromatic essential oils, or the fixed seed and nut oils. The essential oils are distilled from flowers, leaves, peels, and roots of various aromatic plants. Many books and web sites are devoted to essential oils, and for good reason, since they smell lovely and have therapeutic properties.

It is the plant world's *other* oils, the seed and nut oils, that are the focus of this book. Vital for health, the fixed oils are used in food and cooking, skin care, paint, lubrication, and medicine. Their qualities and real-world applications vary according to the plants that produce them. Their ubiquitous presence in all aspects of our lives and far-reaching usefulness is what I want to explore.

My purpose in writing this book is to share what I have learned about oils over some eighteen-plus years of working intimately with them. I'll explain why some oils are solid and some liquid, some red or yellow or clear. Why some last a long time, while others get funky quickly. Where they come from, and most importantly, how to best use them.

I've grown to be quite passionate about oils that the plant world produces, but it hasn't always been that way. This love affair developed over years of cooking and using oils. As an herbalist and maker of topical skin care products, I work with oils almost daily. Eighteen years ago, when I began this adventure with herbs and oils, I used just a few: olive, almond, and castor for the herbal salves, plus coconut and palm to make soap. Oil's oil, more or less, or so I thought.

Learning the art of herbal infused oils is a natural beginning to herbalism. Salves were fun and easy; different combinations of herbs macerated in olive oil made ointments for a variety of conditions. For a time, I infused every kind of plant matter I could get my hands on: chili peppers, eucalyptus leaves, evergreen boughs, pine, cypress, and fir, lichens, flowers like jasmine and roses, along with the usual herbs such as comfrey, calendula, St. John's wort, lemon balm—the list goes on.

In time I became proficient at making creams, by emulsifying oils and watery materials like hydrosols and aloe using beeswax. And soap is pure alchemy, liquid oils turning into hard bars of lather. I loved learning all the techniques and tricks of my craft.

People inquired about classes and I began to teach a few. They were interested in the how of soap, creams and salves. It was in one of these early classes that a student remarked rather casually, "Oh, you must know all about the 'drying' oils."

Huh? I wasn't sure what she was referring to. What dried: The oil? The skin? The oil on the skin? The skin under the oil? As I was in the middle of a class, I nodded noncommittally and continued teaching. But that one remark got me thinking, what on earth did she mean? And I felt a bit silly that I didn't know something that sounded like basic knowledge. I thought I knew my materials pretty well. The question of what a drying oil was stayed with me.

Up to that point, I thought oils were either liquid or solid, unsaturated or saturated, but I hadn't considered dry. Over a period of time it dawned on me that yes, some oils do dry! Think paint. I was carried back to my days in art school, when I had painted with oil paint. It seems an obvious link, but I hadn't considered it—and didn't they add driers to the paint to make it dry?

In time, the phenomena of drying oils began to fall into place. I remembered I had experienced oils "drying" in cooking. Years before, while changing my diet from traditional western fare to a more healthful semi-vegetarianism that eliminated butter, I switched to vegetable oils. Baking projects inevitably require the cook to grease a pan, and liquid oils replaced butter in my kitchen. When resinous and dark brown spots appeared on the pan after the cookies were done, I tried to scrub them off but they wouldn't budge. It was years before I understood why.

As my work with plants continued, understanding the materials I was working with became increasingly important. New oils, such as hazelnut, were added to my repertoire. Hazelnut oil was said to be astringent, a good quality to use on the skin. And I added rose hip seed oil, because it helps heal scar tissue. Then, on a trip to Hawaii, I discovered tamanu, an oil from Tahiti and the Pacific basin. This oil was dark green, nutty smelling, and very healing to the skin. It was said to treat leprous skin lesions! This would be a big plus in a salve.

My soap-making, too, evolved with my increasing awareness of the properties of oils. I added a new range of oils to make better-quality soaps, such as palm kernel oil, used for lather and added hardness. Olive, hazelnut, and other liquid oils would balance the saturated coconut and palm oils to make great skin care bars. If oil lapped at my toes when I began this adventure, I was now up to my knees in it.

As a kinesthetic person, I learn by hands-on activity, and retain information by writing about it. For information to sink in, I must transform it into action or activity. A bar of soap is not just a bar of soap but a lesson plan and exam in one. So too, a salve or study paper make up a curriculum, a process of imprinting and retention that leads ultimately to understanding.

By 2000, I had accumulated so many bits of useful information on oils that I wanted them in one place. I wanted a reference manual where the information would be readily available and easily accessible. Since there wasn't anything that I could find published, I put together a study paper, in the form of a self-published booklet on oils. There were three versions, each adding more information over a two-year period.

The research for this undertaking included my own experiences, published books, and a budding internet. A chemist friend helped me understand the science of making soap. This lead to understanding the structure and basic chemistry of oils, fatty acids, triglycerides, saturated, unsaturated, polyunsaturated, and finally, the drying oils! The phenomena of oils drying finally clicked, and I could now understand the chemistry of what happens when some oils dry and others don't. I had come to the point where I was able to answer the question asked of me by my student years before. I used those first study books as reference material for years.

I continued to use more and different kinds of oils in my work. Sesame became my preferred oil for herbal extractions, instead of olive, the herbal world's standard. It wasn't as oily feeling and helped the quality of my products, especially the creams. Organic oils became more available and affordable and I moved in that direction. Exotic-sounding oils, not necessarily organic, began being listed by my suppliers. Just what were these newer oils?

In 2012, I was invited back to California to teach a class on making creams and herbal emulsions. We had moved up the coast to the Pacific Northwest in 2004. I was asked whether I could bring copies of my original booklet on oils with me to offer to the class.

After ten years, all copies of the booklet had been sold or given away. Additional years of work with the oils had added significantly to my knowledge base. The booklet needed revision and additional content. I had gained greater understanding of the chemistry and structure of oils, and clarification of the original content was necessary. A complete re-write was begun. Originally thirty-six pages, the booklet grew to over eighty pages. The original thirty-five oils profiled turned into seventy, then eighty, different oils. Oil descriptions and fatty acid tables were expanded, while various lists and reference material were also added.

Researching and rewriting renewed my enthusiasm for the subject. By now, my oil immersion had moved from my knees to somewhere around my mid-section. The first booklets centered around the chemistry and structure of the oils, but there was so much more to them. Color, texture, taste, functional properties, and use—surely those qualities had to be addressed too, as my new research lead deeper into the world of oils.

A large part of the research was experiential. I ordered sample sizes of new and exotic oils and relished their different colors: reds, green, all shades of yellow, and clear white. By physically experiencing them, I understood each oil better. I began a daily ritual; at the end of my bath I took a small amount of one oil in my hands and rubbed it into the wet skin on my arms, neck, and face to get the feel of the oil of the day. Unsurprisingly, every oil is a different experience. My head knew this, but now my body could feel the differences in texture, scent and weight.

Unique in their signature properties, oils had personalities that reflected their botanical species and geographical origin. They smelled and felt differently from each other; some soaked in while others sat on the skin. Some formed a whitish film with the water, while others didn't. Some could be felt on the skin all day, others seemingly gone within mere minutes. Experiencing the variety and range of qualities presented new puzzles to unravel and questions to be answered.

What you have in your hands is the culmination of the experiential learning, the researching and questioning. Knowledge is cumulative. This is what I have learned and experienced to date, and no doubt the learning will continue.

I envision this book being useful for those who like to make products, those who work with plants and herbs, massage therapists, aestheticians, soap-makers, and anyone else with an interest in the subject. It is my hope that those who work with oils and want to understand their materials in greater depth will find this work helpful and a good beginning to their own research.

Let's Look at the Lipids

Comforting on both the skin and in the stomach, oils fill us up and protect our hides. We appear more beautiful, our dryness banished and fine lines filled in, the skin's moisture plumped and protected. The ancients regularly oiled their bodies, as did Cleopatra, that ancient symbol of womanly beauty.

Before the age of running water and daily baths, cleansing consisted of removing the previous day's oil and reapplying more. Oils helped protect the skin from high temperatures and dry air. In northern climates, heavier animal fats replaced vegetable oils for a greater degree of protection from very cold temperatures.

Now that we're emerging from the low-fat diet mania, new studies are rediscovering the natural place of oils and fat. Eating a generous amount of high quality fat and oil on a daily basis can actually keep body weight down, by providing flavor and fullness to satisfy the appetite. Along with a low-carbohydrate, high-vegetable, and moderate-protein intake, dieting to loose weight can be a thing of the past. What is most interesting is the place that fats and oils play in our health on both sides of the skin. They are more than important—they are vital, the fuel for life.

With the prominent role of oils in the health of both skin and internal body functions, understanding their structures and composition gives us oil smarts. That allows us to pick the best oil for the task at hand. Most oils can be used for cooking and skin care, but others will make you intensely ill if consumed. Some oils act as medicine externally, but are less than pleasant when taken internally. Other oils can be used for all three categories: food, medicine, and skin care.

A definition of oil from Wikipedia:

> *An oil is any neutral, nonpolar chemical substance, that is a viscous liquid at ambient temperatures, and is immiscible with water but soluble in alcohols or ethers. Oils have a high carbon and hydrogen content and are usually flammable and slippery. Oils may be animal, vegetable or petrochemical in origin, and may be volatile or nonvolatile.*

A mouthful that sums up oil in a few words. If the forgoing is a bit opaque or only somewhat understandable, follow along with me and you'll soon understand it all. Oils, good and bad, essential and fixed, saturated and unsaturated, used for food and body care, for fuel and in industry, play an essential part in all areas of our lives.

Terms: What is Essential?

Essential oils, essential fatty acids, essential nutrients, flower essences: what do these terms mean and are they interchangeable? *Essential* is a word bandied about to the point of losing its meaning. Used as an adjective, *essential* can be used freely, but when it is a proper or descriptive name it must be applied accurately or the meaning is lost. Terms to distinguish and name natural compounds, including oils, require correct usage for a full understanding of the subject.

Essential is most misused or confusing when it names substances. When something pertaining to our health, the plant's health, or the plant's nature is considered essential because it defines a quality or compound, it is part of its proper name. Words and terms matter. The following are examples of the word *essential* used correctly and otherwise.

The *essential nutrients* are the substances that our bodies must consume in the form of food to thrive. These include the vitamins, minerals, proteins, oils, air, water, and light. When speaking or writing about oils, the term *essential* is often misapplied to include all the important and healthful oils. There are however, only *two essential fatty acids* found in oils, which will be discussed later. As important as all the fatty acids and the oils that contain them are, they can be made in the body or derived from the two that are considered *essential*.

Example 1: *Oils are essential in the diet.* This is a true statement and proper use of the word "essential." Example 2: *Olive oil is one of the essential oils for health.* Essential, in this sentence, implies that olive oil is an essential nutrient, that it must be consumed. Olive oil is valuable and healthful, but it's not *essential*, since it could be replaced by a number of other similar oils. Example 3: *Olive oil is essential for Italian cooking.* With this substitution the phrase is now true. Terms and how they are used matters.

Essential oils, however, are a completely different form of plant compound than the oils and fatty acids found in the seeds. Often aromatic, and functioning as messenger molecules, they are considered the *essence* of the plant, its life blood. Here, the term *essential* refers to the compounds' importance to the parent plant. They are not necessary for human health, but we derive great pleasure and benefit from them. They are *essential* compounds for the plants that create them.

Flower essences, in contrast to the essential oils, are energetic remedies made from flowers. Often confused with the *essential oils* because of the similar name and association with flowers, these are not extractions of compounds from the plants. Rather, they are a capturing of the energetic imprint, the healing vibrations of the flower, which is their essential, non-physical nature. Preserved with alcohol and without scent, these remedies are used to gently influence the emotional state of an individual.

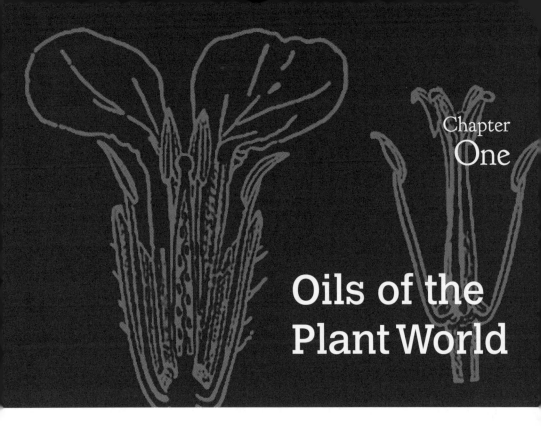

Oils of the Plant World

Oils are of two general types: living oils from growing plants and animals, and the petrochemical oils. *Petra,* the Greek word for rock, the root of petroleum, refers to oil produced from organic matter so ancient it has become like rock. The petroleum oils are better suited to industry than use on the body, and are well-represented and researched by the petrochemical industry. Here, I'll discuss oils from the plant world.

The natural living oils mimic the oils our own bodies make, and include compounds to nourish and protect skin cells. The plant kingdom spans every region on earth, with the exception of the Arctic, and only the extreme polar regions are devoid of oil-producing plants. There, humans rely on animal fats for their health and longevity. The rest of us, however, have a mind-bogglingly wide variety of oils to choose from.

Nonvolatile oils, oils that are fatty and fixed and don't evaporate, are edible and culinary, burnable in lamps or candles, sensual and protective as skin care. They are produced from seeds. For our purposes, this includes the nuts, grains, kernels, fruiting bodies, and seeds of all sizes that have the potential to produce the next generation of a plant. Fruiting bodies are parts of seeds like the flesh on olive pits and the soft fruit of avocados. Both olives and avocados are pressed for oil, and produce two separate oil products. In olives, the various grades of virgin oil comes from the flesh, while pomace oil comes from the pits. In avocados the oil is extracted from either the fruit or the pit. Large as coconuts or as tiny as raspberry seeds, kernels, nuts, fatty fruits, and seeds all have oil-bearing potential.

The other plant-produced oils are the volatile essential oils of aromatherapy, the oils that scent everything from lotions to cleaning supplies. A great number of books and web sites have been devoted to exploring these oils. They too come from the plant world, but from different parts of the plant. We'll look at how they differ from the nonvolatile oils. First, a preview of our primary subject: the nonvolatile fixed oils.

Lipids and the Fixed, Carrier, and Base Oils

As whole substances, oils are made of various compounds specific to their botanical source. The word oil comes from the French *oile* and Latin *oleum,* which in turn comes from the Greek word for olive, *elaion.* Each type of oil is a totality, a wholeness that is different from all other oils. Almond oil, pressed from the nuts of the almond tree, is made up of characteristic components in proportions that are specific and unique to almonds. With small variations dependent on seasonal, regional, and varietal conditions, almond oil is the sum total of what almonds bring to the pressing. The same picture can be painted for olives or sunflower seeds.

All oils are lipids, but not all lipids are oils. *Lipids*, a term from the Greek *lipos* for fat, is the main component (95% to 99%) of an oil. All lipids are made up of the same fundamental building blocks, fatty acids, and triglycerides.

(The section on chemistry will go into more detail on lipid structure.)

Present throughout nature, lipids are created by both animals and plants. Oils provide energy and nourishment for germination to take place in the seeds, nuts, and kernels of plants. As stored energy from sunlight, the nutrition necessary for reproduction produces an incredibly wide array of oils. Plant oils produce high-quality lipids as well as nourishing compounds, including proteins, waxes, vitamins, minerals, antioxidants, and the tocopherols, plus chlorophyll, phytosterols, squalene, and other non-lipid nourishment for the germinating seed.

The oils that are the primary subject of this book are usually described by the names fixed, carrier, and base. The large molecules of these oils do not evaporate like the smaller, volatile essential oil molecules. They are *fixed*, non-evaporating, oils. Because essential oils are strong compounds and are not used straight on the skin, they are diluted in *base* oils, which are *fixed*, and act as *carriers* for the essential oils.

These nonvolatile oils have substance: they are oily or fatty, solid or liquid. The seeds, nuts, and kernels of the plant kingdom are pressed, often under pressure, extracting the oil, which is then filtered and refined in some way before use. Fixed oils can be single crop products, where the plant is grown exclusively to produce oil, or a by-product of food production. Olive and sunflowers are single crop oil producers, while newer oils like raspberry, blueberry, or tomato seed fall into the category of oils produced after other parts of the fruit have been removed.

Oil or fat: when solid fats are melted, they are like liquid oils. The differences between fats and oils is their structure and source, rather than their chemistry. Fats are often solid and animal, while oil is liquid and vegetable. Vegetable oils can be liquid or solid, whereas animal fats are solid. The solid vegetable oils are often called butters, as in mango or shea butter, but are still classified as oils.

Most importantly, fats and oils are vital building blocks of living organisms, our cells being 50% fat and our brain 60%. As part of every cell's structure, fats are integral to life processes and enable the incredibly complex biological functioning of the body. Nature is not on a *low-fat* diet, and certainly not a *no-fat* one.

While researching oils from around the world, I discovered that the respect, even sacred regard, for the trees and plants that produce native oils is palpable. Local names given to the oils often include the words gold or life: *Liquid Gold, Gold of Pleasure, Tree of Life, Green Gold*, or just a respectful *Oil Tree*. In Tahiti, the tamanu tree is worshiped; the local gods are seen sitting in its branches watching the events of life below. In the Middle East, Mohammed considered the tiny seeds of nigella as the source of health, able to cure any condition except death! Worldwide, oils play a large role in maintaining the health and well-being of every culture and community.

Industry also uses plant-sourced oils. Traditional uses of lamp oils like Hawaii's *kukui*, or candlenut, for light have evolved into a staggering range of products and applications. Modern manufacturing uses oils for many different purposes, including paint and flooring, and increasingly as fuel for biodiesel-powered vehicles.

Oils are truly the basis for life. Whether used in sacred ritual or secular application, they are central to our lives. This book's purpose is to explore plant-based oils with an emphasis on topical use and benefits for the skin. But first, let's look at the other oils from plants, the aromatic essential oils.

Essential Oils

Essential oils are also oil products of the plant kingdom. Their volatile compounds disburse into the air, releasing aromas as they evaporate. Complex scented compounds define and identify each plant variety, from lavender to lemon, rose to rosewood. They are considered the life blood of the plant.

Essential oils are not included with the lipids, the fixed oils, as their chemical structure is different. Scent and volatility, the primary characteristics of the essential oils, contrast with the fatty, oily substance of the fixed oils.

The aromatic plants produce volatile compounds in specialized glands. The source of these glands is not localized in any one part of a plant, and includes leaves and flowers, roots, bark, peels, wood, resins and gums. Some seeds are also aromatic. They can be pressed for fixed oils or distilled for their aromatic compounds. The carrot seed, *Daucus carota,* is one such seed.

The role these aromatic compounds play in the life of plants is not fully understood. Some contribute to the plant's immune system, while others are considered the end product of plant metabolism. The complexity of the compounds making up essential oils is staggering. Consisting of several hundred to thousands of organic chemicals, the plants produce these chemical messengers for reasons of their own. Despite on-going research, we may never fully grasp the whole picture of the role they play in the parent plant.

The aroma chemicals include antioxidant actions that help protect the plant, along with antiseptic, anti-inflammatory, anti-bacterial, anti-fungal, and anti-parasitic compounds. These aromatic compounds attract insects, animals, and humans, furthering reproduction.

Various extraction methods are used to separate the volatile oils from the plant material, with steam distillation the most common. This process uses a closed container, in which steam is allowed to permeate the plant material, volatilizing the plant's aroma compounds. These compounds are re-condensed and captured before evaporating, with the lighter volatile essential oils floating on the surface of the distillation water. The distilled water, now called hydrosol, is drawn off from below. Many plants have some aromatic compounds, but not all are subjected to the distillation process.

The essential oils are removed for aroma uses and the water, now a plant-impregnated hydrosol, can be used for skin care, household use, or even in cooking. In the Middle East, rosewater and orange flower waters delicately scent traditional dishes. Lavender water or hydrosol is used to launder fine linens and calm jagged nerves.

Not all plants release their precious oils and scents to steam, and other methods of extraction are also used. Solvents, often alcohol or fat (used in enfleurage), produce absolutes or concretes, aroma compounds that are used in ways similar to the essential oils. Carbon dioxide, CO_2, is also used in yet another more modern method of extraction that produces essential oils and concretes without the use of heat.

The quantity of volatile compounds in a plant varies widely species by species, and the cost of essential oils varies widely on the market. For this reason, some oils sell at wholesale prices for as little as a few dollars an ounce, while the rare and exotic scents like rose or melissa (lemon balm) can sell for many hundreds of dollars an ounce for the pure undiluted oil.

Volatile essential oils carry healing properties from the plants, with the therapeutic properties varying according to the chemical makeup of the individual plants. Used in creams, salves, scrubs, oils, or soap, the beneficial properties are delivered topically to the skin. Aromatherapy, the modern discipline of treating the body with essential oils, was developed in France and includes a notable medical textbook published in 1990, *L'aromatherapie exactement* by Pierre Franchomme and Daniel Penoel. The volume combines modern scientific principles with an aromatic and holistic approach to treatment.

Fragrance oils, unlike true essential oils, are synthetically created scents. They are inexpensive and chemically consistent, making them attractive to the cosmetic industry. Fragrance oils, however, have no health-supporting or therapeutic benefits. Being synthetic, they can also build up in the sensory organs and cause allergies and sensitivities.

Spiritual Nature of Oils

If the material plane has an archetypal source in the spiritual realm, then oils represent the quality of spiritual warmth. In *Healing Plants: Insights Through Spiritual Science,* Wilhelm Pelikan attributes the spiritual element of warmth to oils, both essential oils and fixed oils. On the material plane, the fixed and essential oils are not related, but from this broader viewpoint they represent extremes of a polarity.

Warmth, in this context, is of an idealized, archetypal quality, not the actual heat from a fire. Existing on a plane of mutual opposition, of polarity, the quality of warmth is expressed on one hand as volatility and on the other as substance. Both essential oils and fixed oils embody warmth on opposing sides of the spectrum.

The fixed oils are fatty and oily, expressing the element of spiritual warmth as substance. They are oils that are used to light our nights and heat our food. They are olive or coconut, sunflower or cocoa butter. The opposing pole is volatile, aromatic, dispersing, giving off and evaporating. Being airborne, the volatile oils reach our noses and we smell them. They are the plant scents, the essential oils of aromatherapy, represented by aromatic oils like lavender or lemon.

In other words, opposing poles of warmth share the quality differently. Physicality, fixed, oily, and fatty on one hand; volatile, diffusive, aromatic on the other. Concentration verses dispersion; earthly verses atmospheric.

Chemically, the fixed oils are long chains of carbon molecules; bent, angled, or straight, they are heavy and fatty. They stain paper and cloth with oily smears and they can remain either fatty and solid or dry into a tacky viscous state. They maintain their physical presence; these are the lipids.

On the opposite pole, the compounds of essential oils are composed of very short carbon chains of low viscosity and low vapor pressure, resulting in the volatility of these molecules. The low viscosity and vapor pressure causes these oils to evaporate, allowing the scents to readily disperse into their surroundings. These are the essential oils of aromatherapy, and are not lipids.

Regional Differences in Oil-Bearing Plants

The plant kingdom is represented everywhere except at the polar extremes. East and west, north and south, seeds are produced and many are pressed for oil. Growth patterns in different climates produce different types of oils. Regional conditions influence the properties of oils, with northern latitudes producing oils far different than those grown at the equator.

In the temperate regions of the northern or southern hemispheres, growing conditions vary with seasonal changes that include often-extreme variations of day length and temperature. Plants grown in temperate regions have greater influences associated with the poles and the sun.

Plants grown in temperate regions produce liquid, unsaturated oils. These oils are considered *active*, with a greater affinity to oxygen, than their counterparts in the equatorial regions. The forces associated with the polar extremes, including the day length and seasonal variations, produce oils that can take up oxygen in their carbon chains. These are the oils that must be protected from going rancid, such as flax, walnut, or chia seed oils.

In the tropics at the equator, plant growth is fundamentally different. Roots drop down to the ground from branches high up in trees, flowers and fruiting pods grow outward from trunks and branches, palms and non-deciduous trees proliferate. These unrelenting growth patterns have greater earth forces than polar forces, with little seasonal change or temperature variations.

The warmth and abundant vegetative growth of the tropics and semi-tropics produce hard and semi-hard vegetable butters and oils. These saturated oils cannot easily carry oxygen in their molecular structure. The hard saturated oils resist rancidity and are stable under a variety of conditions.

Tropical oils also contain a greater degree of natural sun-screening components than their temperate cousins. This particular gift from nature in places where the sun is most intense is a welcome attribute. Being saturated and solid, these oils are emollient and protective. They aren't absorbed into the skin layers as easily as liquid oils, and form a protective barrier that slows moisture loss from the skin and body. Examples are coconut, cocoa butter, shea, and mango butter.

Oils in Human Culture

In traditional cultures, it is usually the women of the tribe who collect and process the nuts and kernels to make the oils for their families and communities. Oils fall into the realm of the domestic arts of cooking, body and hair care, child and infant care, candle making and lamp tending, soap making and traditional medicine. Oils and scent are also traditional tools of the womanly arts, including seduction. Cleopatra oiled her body with sweet-scented oils for protection against a harsh environment, as well as to seduce Mark Antony.

Used for industrial purposes and manufacturing, oil becomes the masculine lubrication of culture and moves out of the domestic realm, away from the hearth. The collection and refining of great quantities of oil transforms it into an active part of the invention and alteration of the environment. Oils are used for the lubrication of machinery and the making of paint and lacquers, flooring, and a wide range of modern materials.

Anointing oils are featured in stories throughout the Bible and ancient texts. Olive oil was considered sacred in the Mediterranean, and as an anointing oil it was used to confer an exalted status on people, objects, or buildings. First blessed by the priest, then poured or applied to the subject being anointed, blessings were transferred from the Divine to the commonplace, thereby consecrating and making holy the person or object. Oils in some traditional cultures are revered and considered the dwelling place of the gods. In India, sesame oil is used extensively in Ayurvedic philosophy and practices.

Just what are these magical, special, and vital substances from nature?

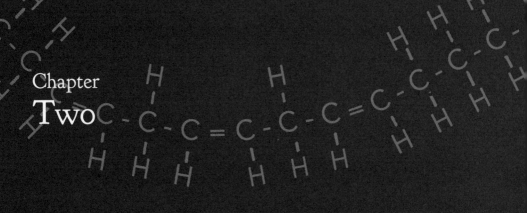

Chapter Two

Lipid Structure and Chemistry 101

The Structure of Fixed Oils

Oils are products of nature and as such, each plant produces oils unique to its species. Similarities occur within botanical families and geographical regions, but ultimately each type of oil is specific to its source. However, all oils are similar in structure and made up of two parts. The major component (85 to 99%) is the lipids, the combinations of fatty acids. A minor but important part comes from plant compounds that give the oils their individuality, color, taste, and scent. Within this simple description lies a complex and vast variety of combinations.

The chemistry of lipids is an extremely complex subject and far beyond the scope of this text. Yet to understand the oils, and the differences between them, a basic knowledge of their chemistry and structure is important. We'll undertake a little "Lipid Chemistry 101" here, looking at the differences between solid and liquid oils, why some oils dry while others harden but don't dry, what makes oils behave the way they do, and what produces the different colors, textures, and feel on the skin.

Terminology can be useful. As chemical units, oils are *hydro-phobic*, meaning they resist water. They are also *lipo-philic*, meaning they attract other oils and fats. Just as the terms hydro-phobic and lipo-philic mean repelling water and attracting oil, respectively, *hydro-philic* and *lipo-phobic* mean attracting water and repelling oil. Polarity, in chemistry, has to do with affinity to water. Chemically, oils are referred to as non-polar substances, meaning they do not dissolve in water.

Fatty Acids and Triglycerides

Fats and oils, the lipids of animal and vegetable origin, are composed of fatty acids. These are made up of long chains of varying numbers of carbon atoms, with hydrogen atoms attached to most or all of the carbon atoms. The variety of patterns of the hydrogen attachment creates the qualities that make up the numerous types of fatty acids, and ultimately oils. **Fatty acids** are the building blocks of oils.

The **carbon chains** of fatty acids can vary from just a few carbon atoms up to twenty-four or more. The lengths of the chains have a great deal to do with the qualities the fatty acid brings to the oil. Yet every oil is a combination of multiple lengths of carbon chains, from short to medium to long and very long. This is where some of the variety happens. It's all in the patterns that nature has devised.

Fatty acids are the basis of **triglycerides.** Three, *tri-*, fatty acid molecules attach to one glycerol, a glyceride molecule. The form looks much like a upper case E, as shown below.

Lipid = Triglyceride = 1 glycerol molecule + 3 fatty acid molecules

The glycerol molecule is the backbone of a triglyceride. Imagine a three-fingered hand with the fingers being the fatty acids joined to a glycerol "palm." Both saturated and unsaturated fatty acids can be found on a single glycerol molecule, the "fingers" being different sizes, shapes, lengths, and types.

$$
\begin{array}{c}
H \\
| \\
H - C - OH \\
| \\
H - C - OH \\
| \\
H - C - OH \\
| \\
H
\end{array}
$$

The glycerol backbone, the vertical of the E of the triglyceride

The glyceride portion of a triglyceride is made up of a gylcerol molecule consisting of three pairs of carbons with oxygen and hydrogen. An oxygen atom with a hydrogen atom attached is called an hydroxyl group, -OH. Fatty acids attach to each of the three oxygen/hydrogen pairings, the hydroxyl groups, and form a triglyceride. The hydroxyl groups are water-soluble, making glycerol a polar substance. Polar substances are both soluble in, and attracting of, water, meaning they are hydro-phillic.

Glycerol backbone **E** with 3 fatty acid molecules attached

Glycerin is a substance that is used in skin care, food products, and industry. The glycerol molecule of a triglyceride is the source of glycerin. Hydroxide ions are used to liberate the fatty acids from the glycerol of triglycerides, forcing them apart to form free fatty acids and glycerin in a process called hydrolysis.

Glycerin is viscous, colorless, and sweet-tasting, 20% heavier than the same volume of water. It has a low glycemic load, being absorbed into the body more slowly than sugar. As a preservative and extracting medium, glycerin is used for making herbal glycerites. In cosmetics and skin care, it is considered a humectant, which means that it draws water to itself, thus helping moisturize the tissues.

Hydrolysis is the chemical process used in making soap. Large commercial soap-makers remove the glycerin for other purposes, or sell it as a by-product. Craft soap-making retains the glycerin due to low-tech methods of production and for its beneficial effects on the skin.

The Carbon Chains

All fatty acids consist of carbon chains, which are carbon atoms linked to each other one after another. We'll attach the hydrogen atoms to these carbon atoms in the next section. The carbon chains have an end that consists of the oxygen and hydroxyl group, oxygen and hydrogen, which makes the chain a fatty acid. This is called a *carboxylic acid* with a long *aliphatic tail*. All fatty acids have a similar structure:

$$- C - C - C - C - C - C - C - C - C - \qquad C = O$$
$$ O\, H$$

aliphatic (non aromatic) *tail,*   carbon chain *carboxylic acid*
(hydrogen atoms not yet attached)   a carboxyl group

Any chain will have two ends and carbon chains are no different. One end is water-soluble and called an acid end (hydrophilic—water loving). It is this end that attaches to the glycerol molecule. The other end is the fatty end and is free, not attached. Being fatty, it is water insoluble (hydrophobic—water repelling), which makes the triglyceride, oil, repel water. Repelling water makes oils, triglycerides, non-polar substances. Again, **polar** means water-attracting, and **non-polar**, water-repelling.

Chemistry is the science of the structure, composition, and transformation of matter. Chemical bonds between atoms are shared electrons that link atoms to form molecules. Carbon atoms always share four electrons with other atoms, and oxygen atoms share two, while hydrogen shares one electron bond. The bonds of the atoms are always the same for carbon, oxygen, and hydrogen.

Hydrogen atoms always have 1 bond with other atoms: H-

Oxygen atoms always have two bonds with other atoms: O=

Carbon atoms always have four bonds with other atoms: =C=

Fatty Acids

Fatty acids come in a variety of forms, saturated, unsaturated, long, short, straight, bent, mono-, poly-, and super-unsaturated. They combine in many different ways, which we will address in the coming sections. These many forms of fatty acids create all the oils produced by nature. Lengths of carbon (C) atom chains from four to twenty-four and above are the molecular building blocks of lipids. Each fatty acid has a name and distinguishing characteristics that makes it different from other fatty acids. There are common fatty acids, such as oleic, found in all oils, and rare fatty acids like punicic acid, found in only a few oils. A few fatty acids play supporting roles in the make-up of many oils, but as very small percentages. Palmitoleic and myristic acids are two such fatty acids.

Isomers in chemistry are molecules that share the same chemical formula, but with a different arrangement of atoms. One example of the formation of fatty acid isomers happens in the digestion of oils. Our metabolic processes take fatty acids from our food and rearrange them into similar, but not identical, fatty acids to create the form the body needs. These are naturally formed isomers. Isomerisation of fatty acids can also occur as a result of high heat or by the process of hydrogenation, and these are unnatural.

Fatty acids are grouped according to the lengths of their (C) carbon chains. **Short-chain fatty acids** have carbon chains of less than eight carbons. **Medium-chain fatty acids** have chains between eight and twelve carbons. **Long-chain fatty acid** chains have lengths of between fourteen and eighteen. Less common are the **very-long-chain fatty acids**, which have twenty carbons and above.

Saturated Oils and Fatty Acids

The solid oils, such as cocoa butter and shea butter, are made up of a high proportion of longer chain saturated fatty acids. Animal fats, too, are for the most part saturated. In a saturated fatty acid chain, the carbon (C) atoms are literally *saturated* with hydrogen (H) atoms. Saturated fatty acids (SaFA) have two hydrogen atoms attached to each of the carbon atoms of the chain.

Each carbon atom has two attached hydrogen atoms.

$$H \quad H \quad H \quad H \quad H \quad H \quad H \quad H \quad H$$
$$| \quad | \quad | \quad | \quad | \quad | \quad | \quad | \quad |$$
$$- C - C - C - C - C - C - C - C - C -$$
$$| \quad | \quad | \quad | \quad | \quad | \quad | \quad | \quad |$$
$$H \quad H \quad H \quad H \quad H \quad H \quad H \quad H \quad H$$

a saturated fatty acid carbon chain

Saturated oils never dry. They remain oily and greasy-feeling to the touch. The solid oils may melt and re-harden but they never become *dry* to the touch. Saturation is directly related to the attraction of atoms to each other. The atoms in the carbon chains do not have any carbon-to-carbon double bonds and they are literally "saturated" with hydrogen atoms. The long, straight, single bond (-) hydrocarbon chains are slow to react chemically, and have no electric charge, no electron activity.

The sharing of hydrogen atoms is called hydrogen binding. Having all the carbon atoms bonded with hydrogen atoms is what creates the saturated solid fats. Due to the hydrogen being bound to each carbon, the saturated fatty acid molecules are straight, without any bend. They are able to pack tightly together into a form that makes them viscous and solid at room temperature. The longer the saturated chain, the higher the melting point and the more solid and hard the fat.

Below is a schematic of nine common saturated fatty acids, four to twenty carbon lengths:

Saturated Fatty Acids; Four to Twenty Carbons long

Butyric Acid (4:0)

```
    H   H   H
    |   |   |
H – C – C – C – C = O
    |   |   |   |
    H   H   H   OH
```

Caproic Acid (6:0)

```
    H   H   H   H   H
    |   |   |   |   |
H – C – C – C – C – C – C = O
    |   |   |   |   |   |
    H   H   H   H   H   OH
```

Caprylic Acid (8:0)

```
    H   H   H   H   H   H   H
    |   |   |   |   |   |   |
H – C – C – C – C – C – C – C – C = O
    |   |   |   |   |   |   |   |
    H   H   H   H   H   H   H   OH
```

Capric Acid (10:0)

```
    H   H   H   H   H   H   H   H   H
    |   |   |   |   |   |   |   |   |
H – C – C – C – C – C – C – C – C – C – C = O
    |   |   |   |   |   |   |   |   |   |
    H   H   H   H   H   H   H   H   H   OH
```

Lauric Acid (12:0)

```
    H   H   H   H   H   H   H   H   H   H   H
    |   |   |   |   |   |   |   |   |   |   |
H – C – C – C – C – C – C – C – C – C – C – C – C = O
    |   |   |   |   |   |   |   |   |   |   |   |   |
    H   H   H   H   H   H   H   H   H   H   H   OH
```

Myristic Acid (14:0)

```
    H   H   H   H   H   H   H   H   H   H   H   H   H
    |   |   |   |   |   |   |   |   |   |   |   |   |
H – C – C – C – C – C – C – C – C – C – C – C – C – C – C = O
    |   |   |   |   |   |   |   |   |   |   |   |   |   |
    H   H   H   H   H   H   H   H   H   H   H   H   H   OH
```

Palmitic Acid (16:0)

```
    H   H   H   H   H   H   H   H   H   H   H   H   H   H   H
    |   |   |   |   |   |   |   |   |   |   |   |   |   |   |
H – C – C – C – C – C – C – C – C – C – C – C – C – C – C – C – C = O
    |   |   |   |   |   |   |   |   |   |   |   |   |   |   |   |
    H   H   H   H   H   H   H   H   H   H   H   H   H   H   H   OH
```

Stearic Acid (18:0)

```
    H   H   H   H   H   H   H   H   H   H   H   H   H   H   H   H   H
    |   |   |   |   |   |   |   |   |   |   |   |   |   |   |   |   |
H – C – C – C – C – C – C – C – C – C – C – C – C – C – C – C – C – C – C = O
    |   |   |   |   |   |   |   |   |   |   |   |   |   |   |   |   |   |
    H   H   H   H   H   H   H   H   H   H   H   H   H   H   H   H   H   OH
```

Arachidic Acid (20:0)

```
    H   H   H   H   H   H   H   H   H   H   H   H   H   H   H   H   H   H   H
    |   |   |   |   |   |   |   |   |   |   |   |   |   |   |   |   |   |   |
H – C – C – C – C – C – C – C – C – C – C – C – C – C – C – C – C – C – C – C – C = O
    |   |   |   |   |   |   |   |   |   |   |   |   |   |   |   |   |   |   |   |
    H   H   H   H   H   H   H   H   H   H   H   H   H   H   H   H   H   H   H   OH
```

Melting point is the temperature that will melt oil from a solid state to a liquid, and is determined by the length and saturation of its fatty acid chains. Unsaturated oils have lower melting points than saturated oils, given equal chain lengths. Four to eight carbon atoms long, saturated fatty acids are liquid at room temperature. The fatty acids in milk and butter are in this category. At ten carbon chains, oils are liquid at body temperature. At fourteen carbons and above, oils are solid unless melted with heat.

Unsaturated Fatty Acids

In contrast to saturated fatty acids, unsaturated fatty acids have a bend in the carbon chain where there is a carbon to carbon double (=) bond. The bend makes the fatty acids unable to pack tightly together, and this causes them to act as liquid. They have the same carbon chains as the saturated fatty acids but the hydrogen atoms are arranged differently on the chains.

Unsaturated fatty acids are just that: **not saturated** with hydrogen atoms. There are breaks on the carbon chains where hydrogen atoms are replaced by a double bond between carbon atoms.

$$
\begin{array}{ccc}
 & H & \\
 & | & \\
C - C - C & \\
 & | & \\
 & H &
\end{array}
\qquad
\begin{array}{ccccccc}
 & H & & & & H & \\
 & | & & & & | & \\
- C - C & = & C - C - \\
 & | & | & & | & | & \\
 & H & H & & H & H &
\end{array}
$$

saturated	unsaturated

In unsaturated chains where two hydrogen atoms (H) appear to be missing, they have been replaced by the double bond = between the carbon atoms. Carbon atoms always have four bonds, where they share electrons with other atoms.

At unsaturated points on the chain, two carbon atoms are linked to each other by a double (=) bond. When there is only one hydrogen attached to each of two consecutive carbon atoms, a double bond (=) between the carbon atoms maintains the chain. The carbon atoms share two electrons with each other when hydrogen is absent. With hydrogen present, its electron is shared with the carbon atoms by a single bond (-).

unsaturated fatty acid chain, in the **cis- configuration**

This structure changes the nature of the fatty acid considerably. At the point of the double (=) bond, the chain forms a bend and is no longer straight as in the saturated chain. Fatty acids typically have one, two, or three, and occasionally more, of these double bonds and therefore kinks in their chains.

This is the **cis configuration,** where hydrogen atoms are absent *on the same side* of the carbon chain. This is an important distinction, and is the most common placement of double bonds and hydrogen. The *cis configuration* creates a bend in the unsaturated fatty acid. When there are multiple bent fatty acid chains they do not lie close to each other, creating a less dense substance, and making the fatty acid act as a liquid rather than a solid. The double bond also has a slight negative charge and the molecules repel each other, creating a tendency to spread and move. Oils stay liquid when made up of a preponderance of unsaturated fatty acids.

Monounsaturated Fatty Acids

Monounsaturated refers to a single double bond (=) in the fatty acid chain. Oils of olive, sesame, almond, and avocado are composed of predominantly monounsaturated fatty acids.

Pictured below is a chain of **oleic acid**, OA (C18:1), a monounsaturated fatty acid. Note the double bond replacing hydrogen atoms on one side of the chain, in this case in the middle at the ninth carbon. Monounsaturated fatty acids, or MUFAs, have one double bond and are fairly stable

Omega 9 Oleic Acid

Polyunsaturated Fatty Acids

Polyunsaturated fatty acids have two or more double bonds, which means they are bent at two or more places. The polyunsaturated fatty acid-dominant oils are often of the omega-6 family, and include oils like grape-seed, evening primrose, safflower, and sunflower.

The following chain of **linoleic acid**, LA (C18:2), is a polyunsaturated fatty acid. Note the two double bonds replacing (H) hydrogen atoms on the chain. Polyunsaturated oils are long-chain fatty acids, most commonly 18 carbons long. The first double bond is at the sixth carbon.

Super/Polyunsaturated Fatty Acids

Often grouped with polyunsaturated oils, superunsaturated fatty acids have three or more double bonds. They are bent at each double bond, creating space between them and other fatty acids. Examples of oils high in the superunsaturated fatty acids are hemp, flax, chia seed, and camelina.

A superunsaturated chain of **alpha-Linolenic acid**, LNA or ALA (C18:3), has three double bonds and has six fewer hydrogen atoms. LNA is an omega-3 fatty acid. The first double bond is at the third carbon.

Unsaturated Fatty Acids and Oxygen

Whereas saturated fatty acids are stable, fixed, and solid, unsaturated fatty acids present a new dynamic in the carbon chain. Oxygen atoms can attach to carbon atoms where they are linked by double bonds. This process is called oxidation. When it happens in edible oils, they are called rancid, but in paint, this is called drying.

Time, heat, and proximity to air and light create conditions where oxygen atoms attach to carbon atoms in the unsaturated chain. The attachment of oxygen causes the once-loosely packed and liquid chains to revert to an inert state that is not subject to further oxidation. The carbon atoms are now bound to oxygen, and the oil containing them becomes not just solid but dry to the touch.

Monounsaturated fatty acids are the most stable of the unsaturated group. Each additional double bond in a fatty acid increases its affinity to oxygen and makes it more and more susceptible to becoming rancid.

The schematic diagram below represents the complex chemical reaction that takes place when unsaturated fatty acids become rancid and oxygen atoms attach to what were double bonds of carbon atoms.

unsaturated chain   oxygen (O) attaches to the carbon atoms

Unsaturated oil is less stable than saturated oil, because it is vulnerable to oxidation in the presence of heat, light, and air. When unsaturated oils oxidize or "dry" they change their molecular structure irreversibly and they can't melt or become "un-dry." To prevent oxidation, oils need protection. They need to be used quickly or refrigerated. Cold temperatures slow the process of oxidation and freezing can stop it altogether, maintaining their quality.

Unsaturated fatty acids can have one double bond, or up to five or more. The most common unsaturated fatty acids are the **Mono,** with one double bond; **Polyunsaturated**, with two double bonds; and **Superunsaturated**, with three or more double bonds. As their state of unsaturation increases, their vulnerability to oxidation increases as well. There are exceptions, but as a rule this is true.

The Ends of the Carbon Chains

Fatty acid chains come in a variety of lengths and degrees of saturation. With the differences and variety in the chains themselves, the ends of fatty acid carbon chains are uniformly all the same. The two ends of opposing poles give fatty acids in oils their unique properties as lipids.

The acid end of the chain is water-soluble (hydrophilic—water loving) and known as a carboxyl (-COOH) group. The fatty end is water-insoluble (hydrophobic—water hating) and ends in a methyl (-CH3) group. This end is also called the omega end.

Fatty End	the (C) carbon chain	**Acid End**
fat soluble		water soluble
water insoluble		fat insoluble
Lipophilic		Hydrophilic

$$H-C \quad C-C-C-C-C-C-C-C \quad -C=O$$

Methyl Group	Variable length	Carboxyl Group
(-CH3)	2 to 26 Carbon chain	(COOH)
Omega (w) free end		Delta (d) end
		attaches to the glycerol

The water-loving, acid ends of all fatty acids attach to the glycerol "palm" of the triglyceride. The other, unattached, end is fatty and repels water, the configuration that makes oil oily. The first acid carboxyl group, the delta end, attracts water and attaches to the glycerol. The other free, unattached end, the fatty, methyl, omega end, attracts oil and repels water, and is oily.

Naming Fatty Acids

Shorthand or Coded System of Fatty Acids

A shorthand description of fatty acid chain length and saturation enables a quick assessment of the type of fatty acid being considered. (This section is indebted to Udo Erasmus' *Fats that Heal, Fats that Kill*, p. 23–25). The shorthanded code for Lauric acid is (12:0), meaning that it has twelve carbon atoms and no breaks in its carbon chain. It is saturated.

Saturated fats, with simple and straight carbon chains, have all the carbon atoms hooked to hydrogen atoms. In order to write the shorthand name for lauric acid, a major component of coconut oil, we need to know the number of carbon (C) atoms, which is 12, as is shown below.

$$H-\overset{\overset{\displaystyle H}{|}}{\underset{\underset{\displaystyle H}{|}}{C}}-\overset{\overset{\displaystyle H}{|}}{\underset{\underset{\displaystyle H}{|}}{C}}-\overset{\overset{\displaystyle H}{|}}{\underset{\underset{\displaystyle H}{|}}{C}}-\overset{\overset{\displaystyle H}{|}}{\underset{\underset{\displaystyle H}{|}}{C}}-\overset{\overset{\displaystyle H}{|}}{\underset{\underset{\displaystyle H}{|}}{C}}-\overset{\overset{\displaystyle H}{|}}{\underset{\underset{\displaystyle H}{|}}{C}}-\overset{\overset{\displaystyle H}{|}}{\underset{\underset{\displaystyle H}{|}}{C}}-\overset{\overset{\displaystyle H}{|}}{\underset{\underset{\displaystyle H}{|}}{C}}-\overset{\overset{\displaystyle H}{|}}{\underset{\underset{\displaystyle H}{|}}{C}}-\overset{\overset{\displaystyle H}{|}}{\underset{\underset{\displaystyle H}{|}}{C}}-\overset{\overset{\displaystyle H}{|}}{\underset{\underset{\displaystyle H}{|}}{C}}-C=O$$
$$OH$$

Lauric acid (12:0)

There are no double bonds (=), so the shorthand name is (12:0). See the diagram of additional saturated fatty acids previously shown.

The same system is used for the unsaturated fatty acids, with the number of double bonds after the colon. The number of carbon atoms in the chain and the number of double bonds creates the following formula (C___:__). Oleic acid is a monounsaturated acid with a code of **C18:1**. C stands for carbon, and 18 for the number of C atoms in the chain. The one (:1) means that it is a mono, single, unsaturated fatty acid.

By comparison, linoleic acid's code is **C18:2**. It is similar to oleic acid in the 18 carbon atoms, but has two double bonds that make it behave differently.

Fatty Acid Names

This section is for reference, and should be useful when confronted with data sheets on oils you may have ordered or researched online. Keep it handy, you never know when you might want it.

Fatty acids have names, but somewhat like people, they have proper names, popular names, and nicknames. As molecules, they also have a molecular structural "name."

The discoverer of a fatty acid often gives it a name based on where it was first found. For example, butyric acid was first found in butter. Arachidic acid is found in peanuts (*Arachis hypogeae* is the botanical name for peanut). Stearic acid is from the Greek root word for fat, which is *stea-*, while palmitic acid was first found in palm oil. Oleic acid, one of the most common fatty acids, is named for the olive.

Unsaturated fatty acids also have carbon chains, but the carbon atoms do not have all of the spaces attached to hydrogen atoms. Instead, the carbon atoms are linked by a double bond (=) where there are missing hydrogen atoms. Our example of an unsaturated fatty acid, linoleic, has two double bonds. The following are some of the names used to describe this fatty acid:

Popular name:

Linoleic Acid

Proper name:

cis- w6, 9-octadecadienoic acid

Shorthand or nickname:

18 : 2w6

The structural formula:

$$H-\overset{\overset{\displaystyle H}{|}}{\underset{\underset{\displaystyle H}{|}}{C}}-\overset{\overset{\displaystyle H}{|}}{\underset{\underset{\displaystyle H}{|}}{C}}-\overset{\overset{\displaystyle H}{|}}{\underset{\underset{\displaystyle H}{|}}{C}}-\overset{\overset{\displaystyle H}{|}}{\underset{\underset{\displaystyle H}{|}}{C}}-\overset{\overset{\displaystyle H}{|}}{\underset{\underset{\displaystyle H}{|}}{C}}-\overset{\overset{\displaystyle H}{|}}{C}=\overset{\overset{\displaystyle H}{|}}{C}-\overset{\overset{\displaystyle H}{|}}{\underset{\underset{\displaystyle H}{|}}{C}}-\overset{\overset{\displaystyle H}{|}}{C}=\overset{\overset{\displaystyle H}{|}}{C}-\cdots$$

Linoleic Acid

The popular name for linoleic acid comes from the Latin name for flax, *Linum*. The explanation for the formal or proper name (*cis*- w6, 9-octadecadienoic acid) is as follows:

❁ *Cis*- means that both hydrogen atoms on the carbon atoms of the double bonds are missing on the **same side** of the carbon chain.

❁ w6, 9 indicates where the double bonds are located, counting from the methyl (w) end. In this case there are two, the first at the sixth carbon and the second at the ninth.

❁ "octadeca" is another way of saying 18 carbons

❁ "di" means two

❁ "en" means double bond

❁ -oic acid means a fatty acid.

The shorthand name, 18:2w6, shows that the first of the two double bonds begin at the sixth place from the **w** (methyl) end of the carbon chain. See the diagram of a basic fatty acid, which shows the fatty (methyl group) Omega (w) end, the carbon chain, and the acid end (carboxyl group). The double bonds of unsaturated fatty acids are always counted from the omega (w) methyl end. Therefore, 18:2w6 means:

- 18 is the number of carbon atoms

- 2 is the number of double bonds

- w6 is the position of the first double bond(s) on the chain.

Omega Classification

Families of fatty acids are classified by their chemical structure. These families relate to the degree of saturation of the oils in the group. Saturated fatty acids are simply called "saturated." The unsaturated oils have "omega" names: omega-3, omega-6, and omega-9 are the most common, and are based on the structure of the fatty acid.

The omega name is determined by the number of carbon atoms from the omega, free end-to the first double bond of the carbon chain. The first double bond occurs at the third carbon in an omega-3 fatty acid. In an omega-9 monounsaturated oil, the double bond occurs at the ninth carbon atom. There are many different omega classifications, including omega 5, omega 7, and even omega 10.

Chapter
Three

Beyond
Fatty Acids . . .

Fatty acids are the largest component of any oil, but never a hundred percent. The different carbon chain lengths—as short as four, or up to 24 or more, with varying degrees of saturation—create a wide range of properties that distinguish the oils from each other. In addition to the fatty acid composition, additional plant compounds create unique oils from each type of seed.

Imagine saturated fatty acids with rigid straight and unbent carbon chains. Compare them to monounsaturated chains with a single bend. Or, polyunsaturated fatty acids with two double bonds that bend with a distinct kink. More highly unsaturated fatty acids, with three or more double bonds, are so bent they appear to curl. The bent chains can't lie flat, and the space between them creates what appears as liquid. The chains move around each other and remain liquid even under extreme cold. It is these combinations that make up the wide range of oils from nature.

When oxygen enters the picture, we see how oxygen atoms can attach to poly and superunsaturated carbon chains and change their nature. An oil dries by going rancid—a good thing if you are a painter but not when dressing a salad. In the presence of light, heat, and air, the polyunsaturated oils change chemically, and become solid over time as they are susceptible to oxygen attachment.

... to Oils

Whole oils possess compounds that are plant-specific and give the oils properties beyond their fatty acid profile. With different colors, tastes, scents, and nutritional elements, oils are complex mixtures of many different compounds, lipid and non-lipid.

Oils contain both fatty acids, the stored sun energy for reproduction, and non-lipid compounds that are necessary for the health and survival of the seedling. The extra non-lipid portion of the oil contains the vitamins, minerals, proteins, waxes, plant sterols, tocopherols, chlorophyll, carotenes, squalene, antioxidants and many additional compounds that make up the **healing fraction**. In scientific and technical language this is called the **un-saponifiable** portion, a term relating to the process of turning oil into soap.

Oils are amazingly malleable substances. Some are broken apart to make plastics and lubricating compounds. Unsaturated oils like flax make paint and flooring. Known as linseed oil for all but food use, flax is an oil that readily combines with oxygen, drying in the presence of air. The polyunsaturated fatty acids polymerize (skin over), which makes them dry to the touch. This drying, oxidation of the fatty acids, is a slow process unless sped up by heat or chemical driers.

Linoleum gets its name from the fatty acids that make up linseed oil:

linoleic, and alpha-Linolenic acids. The fatty acid names, in turn, come from the flax plant, *Linum*. Linoleum flooring is made by combining sawdust and pigments with flax/linseed oil. The high percentage of alpha-Linolenic acid in flax oil combines with oxygen and dries. Spell-check programs will try to "correct" the fatty acid names to "linoleum" as you type!

Linseed oil creates a tough paint layer, enabling paintings to last for centuries with adequate care. Although linseed oil has been used by painters since the Renaissance, some modern artists have adopted different oils. Walnut and poppy seed oils do not yellow as much as linseed oil as they dry. Meanwhile, safflower and sunflower oil varieties have been hybridized to be high in linoleic acid, and are used for drying applications in industry and house paint.

In the kitchen, oils dry all the time. That tacky feel on the outside of an older bottle of cooking oil is oil in the process of drying. When baking, unsaturated oils used to grease the pan dry into brown oil residues baked onto the surface and cannot be washed off easily. This is "dried" unsaturated oil. Better choices for baking include saturated butter, coconut, or palm oils, which don't dry.

The same fatty acids that cause some oils to dry are also useful as nutritional supplements when fresh. Oils like flax, containing the highly unsaturated omega-3 fatty acids, are packaged in dark containers and kept under refrigeration for protection. When not protected, they can go rancid before being consumed, thus damaging health.

Nature has a great capacity to surprise. Of the wide range of oils with polyunsaturated fatty acids, there are some that remain stable for long periods of time, a year or more. Compounds in the unsaponifiable healing fraction protect the fatty acids from oxygen. Natural antioxidants, vitamins A, C, and E, plus minerals and phytochemicals, resist oxidation. Raspberry seed, cucumber seed, and camelina oils are examples of exceptional stability.

Very-long-chained fatty acids too, even those with multiple double bonds, remain stable for extended periods of time. Egyptian moringa and meadowfoam oils are examples, as both have a high percentage of very long carbon chains. Moringa oil, with its 22 carbon saturated chain of behenic acid, is said to have a shelf life of up to five years. These unsaturated and long-chain fatty acid oils are particularly useful for making skin care products that need a reasonable shelf life, longer than just a few weeks.

Comparing Two Oils: Olive and Cocoa Butter

Radically different in texture, use, color, scent, taste, hardness, and geographical source, olive and cocoa butter are two oils that are perfect for a study in contrasts. Completely different from each other but composed of similar compounds in differing quantities and combinations, the oils possess their own unique signature of the shared compounds.

Olive, a popular oil for its rich flavor and health-giving properties, is liquid at room temperature. 70% of the oil is made up of oleic acid, the monounsaturated fatty acid named for olives. It also contains saturated fatty acids, such as stearic and palmitic acids, in quantities of about 15%. These are the fatty acids that solidify when the oil is stored in the refrigerator. Polyunsaturated linoleic acid makes up 12%. Superunsaturated alpha-Linolenic acid makes up half a percent, with traces of additional fatty acids. Olive oil's unsaponifiables, about half to one percent, include squalene and other compounds that give the oil its flavor and other health-giving properties.

Cocoa butter, by contrast, is a very hard saturated oil scented of chocolate. It is too hard to use directly on the skin without being combined with a less saturated oil. Its hardness derives from the high percentage of long-chain saturated fatty acids, stearic and palmitic acids, that make up 65% of the butter. Monounsaturated oleic acid makes up about 30%. In addition, there are traces of polyunsaturated linoleic and alpha-Linolenic acids, along with other less common fatty acids. The unsaponifiable portion of less than 1% is where the chocolate flavor, scent, and healing compounds can be found.

	Olive	Cocoa Butter
Monounsaturated oleic acid	70%	30%
Saturated stearic & palmitic acids	15%	65%
Polyunsaturated linoleic & alpha-Linolenic acids	12.5%	trace
Unsaponifiable portion	.5–1%	<1%

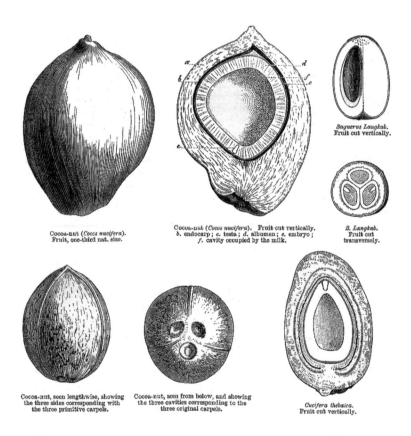

Cocoa-nut (*Cocos nucifera*).
Fruit, one-third nat. size.

Cocoa-nut (*Cocos nucifera*). Fruit cut vertically.
b. endocarp; *c.* testa; *d.* albumen; *e.* embryo;
f. cavity occupied by the milk.

Saguerus Langkab.
Fruit cut vertically.

S. Langkab.
Fruit cut
transversely.

Cocoa-nut, seen lengthwise, showing
the three sides corresponding with
the three primitive carpels.

Cocoa-nut, seen from below, and showing
the three cavities corresponding to the
three original carpels.

Cucifera thebaica.
Fruit cut vertically.

Cocoa Nuts

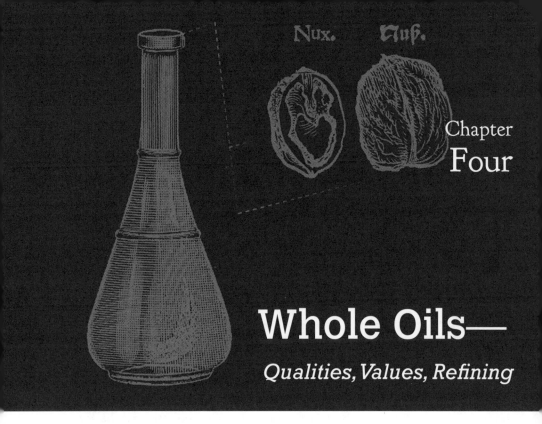

Whole Oils—

Qualities, Values, Refining

Oils exist in the seed for the plant's use, but we must extract the precious liquid or solid fat before we can use them. Once removed from the seeds or nuts, oils are ready for a myriad of uses.

Terms and values have been developed to distinguish between the qualities found in the different oils. Degree of saturation, capacity to turn into soap, weight of the molecules—these, among other qualities, have been reduced to standardized values that simplify information available on oils. Learning to read these values is helpful when working with them.

The refining process too can take many forms. Getting oil from seed to bottle takes many steps by pickers, processers, refiners, distributors, and sellers, each contributing to the final product.

Saponification Value

The process of **hydrolosis** is what turns oils, lipids, into soap. The process of making soap is to saponify oil, transforming it into a new state. Hydroxide ions, lye, break apart the oil's triglyceride structure, creating free fatty acids and glycerin. Through the action of the hydroxide ions, the free fatty acids are transformed into soap.

Each oil has what is known as a *saponification value,* or **SAP value**— the number of milligrams of potassium hydroxide needed to turn the oil into soap. The action of potassium hydroxide, or KOH, on oil makes a soft, almost liquid, soap. For bar soaps hard enough to form and cut, a further calculation is made to determine the correct amount of sodium hydroxide, or NaOH, needed, as sodium creates hardness in soap. The wood ash lime our pioneer ancestors used made a soft soap. To harden it, they added sodium in the form of salt to create bars.

When making soap, the weight and SAP value of each type of oil is calculated to determine the total amount of hydroxide to use for the recipe. Too much lye, and the soap burns or irritates the skin, too little and the soap is spongy and soft, unable to harden into useable bars. A simple internet search will find sites to help in calculating soap recipes. See the appendix for a lengthy list of SAP values for oils.

Unsaponifiable Portion

The lipids, triglycerides, and free fatty acids in oils are the only parts that are transformed into soap molecules by the action of hydroxide ions. The additional plant compounds are called the un-saponifiable portion, meaning they don't saponify and transform into soap molecules. The unsaponifiable portion includes the vitamins, minerals, waxes, polyphenols, and antioxidants, the extra botanical elements that give oils individuality. During the soap-making process, the plant compounds remain in the finished soap unless removed or refined out.

The unsaponifiable portion, also called the healing fraction of an oil, constitutes anywhere from less than 1% to up to 17% of some oils. The term "healing fraction" is not used as often as the more technical term, unsaponifiable fraction. Oils are combinations of similar elements that when combined as a totality are unique in themselves.

Iodine Value of Oils

The *iodine value,* or *iodine index,* determines the degree of saturation of the oil. Remember, oils are made up of a complex combination of fatty acids and triglycerides, both saturated and unsaturated. The number of grams of iodine consumed by 100 grams of a chemical substance, oil in our case, determines its iodine value. The double bonds in the oils' fatty acids react with the iodine compounds, which sets a value for the oil. The more double bonds (=), the higher the iodine value an oil has. For example, linseed/flax oil, which is highly unsaturated, has a value of 170 to 204, whereas cocoa butter, a very saturated oil, has an iodine value of 35 to 40. Olive oil is somewhere in between, with an iodine value of 80 to 88.

Iodine value of three oils for comparison	
Flax/linseed oil	170–204
Olive oil	80–88
Cocoa Butter	35–40

Peroxide Value and Acid Value

The peroxide value of oils measures their degree of rancidity. Peroxide is the primary oxidation product when oil becomes rancid. Unsaturated oils are always in the process of going rancid (oxidizing), as this is part of the chemical process that happens over time. In fresh oils, the oxidation process begins by forming hydroperoxides, a derivative of hydrogen peroxide that is measured by the peroxide value. Very rancid oils have further values that determine their degree of oxidation, but those are not suitable for food or skin care. Data sheets that arrive with bulk oils often include the peroxide value of the oil when it was shipped, and are usually under 2%, and often less than one percent.

The acid value of oils measures the free fatty acids, fatty acids that are no longer combined with their parent triglyceride or phospholipid. This is another method of evaluating the oils that we use and consume.

Fractionation

Fractionation of oil is a natural process where saturated fatty acids within a single oil or mixture of oils clump together and separate from the unsaturated fatty acids. This is sometimes also called crystallization, because the saturated solid fatty acids crystallize and harden. In edible oil processing, fractionation can also be induced by controlled cooling of the oil. The resulting partial crystallization separates the olein, or liquid oil, from the stearin, the solid saturated fractions. Filtering or centrifuging separates the two forms of the oil.

If you store olive oil in the refrigerator, the saturated fatty acids solidify and float in the approximately 85% unsaturated portion. The oil has fractionated into its component parts, but will recombine when the oil is warmed and the saturated fatty acids return to a liquid state. In salve and cream-making, saturated oils can "grow" little lumps that melt with the warmth of the skin. The saturated fatty acids fractionate and coalesce together, causing this state. Keeping temperatures as low as possible when combining and then cooling the product quickly can help reduce this.

Refining Oils

Getting oils from seed to bottle requires a fair amount of processing. First, they must be extracted from the plant material by a variety of methods, either gently by cold processing or less gently by expeller pressing. Solvent extractions are the least desirable extraction process, as the oils' nutritional elements are harmed and solvent residues can remain in the oil.

Once pressed, oil can be simply filtered through clay to remove plant particles and minor impurities. This is the simplest form of refining. Most commercial oils, however, are more highly refined. Once removed from the plant material, the oil can go through up to four processes of refinement to remove color, scent, and other unsaponifiables. The unsaponifiable portion contains beneficial properties that are often refined out of raw oils. These non-lipid extra plant compounds can interfere with quality and shelf life when oils are stored or used for processes that include heat. Highly refined oils store longer, and are less likely to offend by being odorless and colorless. They are characterless as well.

The initials *RBWD* represent the various levels of refining used to prepare oils for the marketplace. The initials stand for *Refining, Bleaching, Winterizing,* and *Deodorizing*.

> **Refining** *involves de-gumming and/or treatment with an alkali to remove phospholipids, sterols, and other natural oil components.*
>
> **Bleaching** *is done with an alkali to neutralize free fatty acids and remove color.*
>
> **Winterizing** *removes natural plant waxes so they don't harden or fractionate in freezing weather.*

Deodorizing *is done by steam distillation under a high vacuum to remove natural plant oil odors.*

One or more of these processes are used on the vast quantity of oils on the market. Shelf life, an important consideration of commerce, is extended by removing unstable elements like free fatty acids. Waxes, scent, and color are removed to create oils that are uniform for the market, ship and store well in all weather, and keep from going rancid too quickly. This is the uninteresting pale vegetable oil found on grocery shelves.

The big players in the cosmetic industry often do not want oils that are full of color and scent, playing up the "purity" of the oils they use. Organic oils, on the other hand, are often lightly refined and retain their natural qualities of color and scent. Batch to batch, oil to oil, organic or commercial, oils of a singular type can vary wildly in quality and properties.

As a personal example, purchasing rose hip seed oil over a fifteen-year span has shown wide variations in color and scent. The organic versions are generally more deeply colored than those commercially grown and processed, but even with the organic products, the color has varied from a light golden to a deep dark orange. These variations could be a product of the crop quality or the refining process or both. Small bottles of oils can usually be ordered for sampling before ordering large quantities.

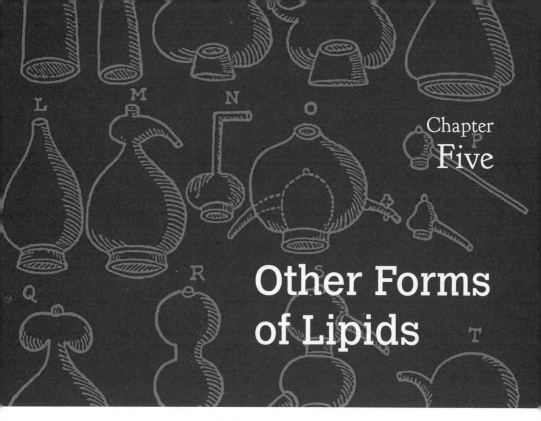

Other Forms of Lipids

Lipids, we now know, consist of fatty acid structures. They can be natural (from plant or animal sources), or chemically altered to create new forms of fatty acids. Phospholipids and waxes are natural forms created by plants and animals for protection and as part of their bodily structures.

Phospholipids—Lecithin

Lecithin is a lipid, a **phospholipid**, with a chemical makeup that's related to triglycerides but different. Phospholipids form a large part of cellular walls in living organisms. A useful ingredient in skin care products because of its skin permeability, lecithin also helps with emulsification.

Phospholipids behave differently from triglycerides because of their different lipid structures. They contain the same glycerol molecule as triglycerides, with the same three points of attachment. But phospholipids have only two fatty acids attached to the glycerol "palm," rather than the three belonging to the triglyceride.

Phospholipid = 1 glycerol molecule + 2 fatty acids
+ 1 phosphate group

The third position on the glycerol molecule contains a *phosphate group*, and that is what makes lecithin able to bridge the world of water and oil. The phosphate group attaches in the third position on the glycerol "palm" and is hydrophilic, meaning that it attracts water. Triglycerides repel water, while phospholipids such as lecithin attract water, to a degree.

Glycerol backbone **F** with 2 fatty acids and a phosphate group

The hydrophilic, or water-loving, properties of the phosphate group cause phospholipids to spread out in thin layers, forming membranes to protect the cells. By forming thin skin-like barriers around cell structures, the nucleus, mitochondria, and lysosomes are protected. These membranes act as barriers to keep what is foreign to the cell out and what is interior to the cell within.

Natural sources of phospholipids include lecithin from egg yolk and vegetable oils, with soybeans the most common source of vegetarian lecithin. All oils contain phospholipids to a greater or lesser degree as part of the unsaponifiable portion of the oil. Phospholipids, with their hydrophilic properties, aid emulsification and skin absorbency. Oils high in lecithin and phospholipids will create a white film on the body when massaged into wet skin and absorb fairly quickly.

Waxes

Waxes are lipids composed of long-chain fatty acids linked by ester bonds to a long-chain alcohol. Alcohols are hydroxyl groups (-OH) bound to a carbon atom. Chemically, waxes differ from oils as they do not contain glycerol molecules or triglycerides. They are extremely hydrophobic, repelling water due to their long, non-polar carbon chains and absence of any hydrophilic glycerol molecules.

Both plants and animals form waxes for protection against moisture loss and as waterproofing. Jojoba "oil" is actually a liquid wax ester produced by the jojoba plant to protect it from the extremes of its native desert environment. Waxes are classified as lipids due to their fatty acid content.

Trans Fats & Oils

Trans fatty acids are fatty acids that have at least one double bond in the trans configuration rather than the more common cis configuration (see page ???). Trans fatty acids can be either natural or synthetically formed. Natural trans fats are found in the meat and dairy of ruminants, such as cows, sheep, and goats. This form is beneficial to health, and called "conjugated fatty acids," as both cis and trans-configured double bonds occur on a single fatty acid chain.

Synthetically formed trans fats are made by altering unsaturated fatty acids through a process called hydrogenation. An industrial process, hydrogenation heats unsaturated oils to high temperatures, often under pressure, in the presence of a catalyst (often nickel). Hydrogen is then introduced and absorbed into the fatty acids, changing the molecular structure into a straighter form from its original bent shape. The normal cis configuration fatty acid chains flip to a trans configuration, creating trans isomers of the original fatty acid form. These are the hydrogenated and trans fats.

Originally developed as a way to use inexpensive unsaturated oils in commercial foods, the partial hydrogenation of oils opened up a large market for many types of foods that had been previously made at home. Baked goods and processed foods became shelf-stable and popular because of changing lifestyle patterns, including availability of preprocessed foods and women increasingly working outside the home. Soybean oil is high in polyunsaturated linoleic acid and accounts for over half the hydrogenated oil in the U.S.

Below is a schematic diagram of a very complex chemical process, representing what happens to liquid unsaturated oils when undergoing the hydrogenation process that transforms them into trans, then fully saturated, fats.

$$
\begin{array}{ccccccccc}
H & H & H & & & & H & H & H \\
| & | & | & & & & | & | & \backslash \\
-C & -C & -C & -C & = C & -C & -C & -C & - \\
| & | & | & | & | & | & | & | \\
H & H & H & H & H & H & H & H
\end{array}
$$

unsaturated chain
Cis-configuration fatty acid
Liquid Natural Oil

$$
\begin{array}{cccccccc}
H & H & \mathbf{H} & & H & H & H & H \\
| & | & | & & | & | & | & | \\
-C & -C & -C & -C & = C & -C & -C & -C & - \\
| & | & | & | & | & | & | \\
H & H & H & H & \mathbf{H} & H & H
\end{array}
$$

Partially hydrogenated
Trans-configuration fatty acid
Margarine/vegetable shortening

$$
\begin{array}{cccccccc}
H & H & H & \mathbf{H} & H & H & H & H \\
| & | & | & | & | & | & | & | \\
-C & -C & -C & -C & -C & -C & -C & -C & - \\
| & | & | & | & | & | & | & | \\
H & H & H & H & \mathbf{H} & H & H & H
\end{array}
$$

fully hydrogenated
no trans fat
waxy like fat for candles

The first diagram is the cis configuration of a natural unsaturated fatty acid, in liquid oil. A sharp kink forms where the double bond is located on the chain in the cis configuration. In the second diagram, the H's represent industrially introduced hydrogen atoms. The chain is no longer sharply bent because in the trans configuration of hydrogen, the double bond does not create such a pronounced kink, and the resulting fatty acid is straighter—closer to a saturated molecule. Partially hydrogenated oils are *"trans-formed"* fatty acid chains. They are called *trans-fatty acids* because the formerly bent, C-shaped *(cis)* polyunsaturated fatty acid is trans-formed into a non-bent semi-saturated fatty acid molecule.

The third diagram represents a fully hydrogenated, and thus saturated, fatty acid where the introduced hydrogen atoms, **H,** have attached to the unsaturated carbon atoms. The single bond replaces the double bond between the carbon atoms in this newly saturated fat. The chain is transformed into a fully saturated fatty acid from an unsaturated one. The result is a wax-like fatty acid that is made into candles but not usually used in food preparation. The melting points of the fatty acids rise with the increased degree of saturation.

Isomers are molecules with the same chemical formula but different arrangements of atoms. In fatty acids there are two forms of isomers, ones that have to do with the geometry of the fatty acid (cis and trans) and the other, where the placement of the double bonds on the carbon chains is what differs. Elaidic acid is the trans isomer of oleic acid of olive oil fame. If oleic acid is fully hydrogenated it becomes stearic acid, which is a hard, waxy fat suitable for candles but not for food. Both fatty acids are C18, eighteen carbon atoms long.

During hydrogenation, the oil is exposed to extremely high pressure and temperatures that degrade the original structure, destroying the essential fatty acids and the fat-soluble vitamins. These laboratory-made fats are a major contributor to diseases of the circulatory system and the heart, and they interfere with the absorption of healthful essential fatty acids in the body. Because these artificial isomers aren't found in nature, the body doesn't recognize them or know what to do with them. Unable to support health, yet widespread throughout the food system, how have trans fatty acids become so popular?

In 1903 the hydrogenation process was developed and patented by a man named William Normann. It was originally intended to create an inexpensive non-animal alternative to tallow for the making of candles, but commercial uses soon expanded. In 1911 Proctor & Gamble—realizing the resulting material looked and behaved like lard, the common cooking fat—created the first vegetable shortening. After branding their product Crisco, the new fat was sold as a substitute for lard.

Hydrogenated fats are cheaper to produce than animal fats, and with the rationing of butter during World War II, the use of margarine and vegetable shortening expanded. Then, in the middle of the twentieth century, a combination of events turned popular opinion against all saturated fats. Urban myth credits the soybean industry with promoting a flawed study which found that saturated fat had caused harm in animal subjects. The misinformation that saturated fats from all sources, both animal and vegetable, were harmful to our health and our hearts in particular was complete. Only in the last few years, with the recognition of the benefits of coconut and other natural saturated oils, and the awareness of the harm from trans fatty acids, has the tide begun to turn back to a more healthful and realistic understanding of these types of fats.

Petrochemicals—Mineral Oil

Mineral oil comes not from minerals but from petroleum, a name from the Greek *petra*, or rock, and the Latin *oleum*, oil. Petroleum is the ancient formation of fossilized organic plants and animal matter. Colloquially called *mineral oil* because its origins are so ancient and rock-like, petroleum is carbon-based because of its plant origins and part of organic chemistry.

Mineral oil is used in many skin care products because of its wide availability and low cost. Considered a non-physiologic lipid (not compatible with normal and healthy functioning skin), petroleum-based mineral oil is incompatible with natural skin care and is not accepted for certified organic skin care products. Unlike living botanical oils, mineral oils do not have fatty acid counterparts in our own skin. They interfere with the absorption of fatty acids that the skin needs while binding with oil-soluble vitamins and hormones in the body. Once bound, nutrients are rendered unavailable as nutrition for the body.

Applying mineral oil to the skin coats it, rather than integrating with the skin's natural oils—a little like wrapping the skin in cling wrap. The skin's natural functions that breathe and interact with the environment are hampered by properties that make mineral oil unsuitable for use in natural skin care products.

Sperm Whale Oil

Sperm whale oil was a popular and sought-after lipid in the eighteenth, nineteenth, and early twentieth centuries. Applications for sperm oil included fuel for lamps and machine oil lubrication as well as skin care. Due to its low viscosity and high stability, it was superior to the oil from other whales, which was composed of less desirable triglycerides. Sperm oil's superior fatty acids and long-chained waxy esters made it sought-after and more expensive in its heyday. It wasn't until the second half of the twentieth century that plant-based alternatives were found and developed as viable replacements.

In the 1970s, jojoba oil was developed to replace the waxy esters found in sperm oil. As a result, liquid waxy esters could be obtained by farming, rather than by killing whales. At a similar point in the 1970s, another crop, meadowfoam, a wildflower native to the Pacific Northwest, was developed as another replacement for sperm oil. Ninety percent of meadowfoam seed oil's fatty acid composition is over 20 carbons long, similar to the waxy esters of jojoba and sperm oils.

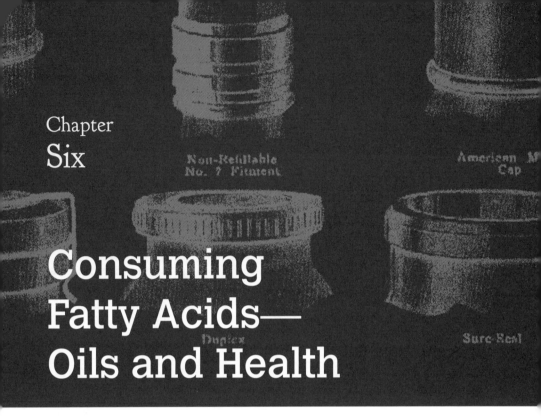

Chapter Six

Consuming Fatty Acids— Oils and Health

Oils are vital for health. As mentioned earlier, our body cells are 50% fat, and our brain cells are 60%. Fats and oils play an important role in maintaining health both inside, through food, and outside, on our skin. Quality fats and oils maintain the integrity of all cells, skin, muscle, bone, and organs. Lipids help the body retain moisture, while oil and waxes protect against the evaporation of water necessary for life to function.

Fats and diet are two words that have become utterly controversial over the past half-century. Poor studies, special interests, misunderstandings, and misinformation conspired to vilify a fundamental food and to manipulate our food choices. In the 1950s a researcher at the University of Minnesota named Ancel Keys began a campaign championing low saturated fat diets as the way to overcome the country's growing heart disease epidemic. Dr. Keys was famously persuasive, eventually landing a position at the American Heart Association, where his flawed premise was made into the dietary guidelines most people follow to this day. Unfortunately his studies were biased and incomplete and have been recently challenged by a study published in the Annals of Internal Medicine in March 2014. Saturated fat is no longer considered bad for us.

With natural forms of saturated fat eliminated from the diet, liquid oils—which were often hydrogenated to preserve them—and carbohydrates took their place. This caused new problems with our national diet to surface. Obesity and diabetes increased and heart disease stayed stubbornly high. In the 1980s the National Institute of Health convened studies to find out why health outcomes from the dietary guidelines hadn't materialized. They were unsuccessful. The dietary guidelines that the country adopted had in fact increased diseases it was supposed to halt and added new ones to the landscape.

Then in the 1990s, no doubt because of the poor showings in our national health, all fats were said to be bad for our health. Low-fat became the standard, and fat calories were replaced with carbohydrates and sugars. Fat imparts flavor to foods, and with its removal, sugars became flavor-carriers necessary to make food palatable. With the launch of the anti-fat craze, rates of obesity and cancer began to climb steadily.

Fat became the enemy instead of a food that sustains and warms our bodies. Triglycerides found in fats from plants and animals in the form of oils and butters make up approximately 95% of all necessary dietary fats. With the propaganda against fat of any kind so successful, surveys showed that in the minds of many individuals fat was considered toxic. Such a sad state for a life-giving product of nature. It will take years to dispel the misinformation that has been perpetuated.

Is fat bad for us? Quite simply, it depends on the kind of fat we eat. Our cells and bodies recognize what nature produces. They are, however, unable to recognize the manipulated, hydrogenated, overheated, chemically extracted oils that are no longer elements of the natural world. When these types of fats are consumed, the body must either eliminate them or store them away, since they don't function as nutrition.

Healthy body functioning relies on all the necessary nutrients, including the essential fatty acids. Natural or organic oils that are minimally refined, stored properly, and used wisely maintain the health of body and skin. Natural oils speak the language spoken by our cells.

In time, the poor studies have been rebuked but the myths live on to this day. This book is designed to give you, the reader, information on the properties and qualities of oil and fats. With knowledge and understanding, you can determine which oils to use and when. For cooking, the saturated oils are best, as they are resistant to damage from heat. For instance, coconut oil has become popular as cooking oil. Natural palm oil is used as shortening in baked goods, replacing the lard of the nineteenth century and the hydrogenated Crisco of the twentieth. Monounsaturated oils, such as olive and sesame, are best used in low-heat cooking and for dressing foods, while the nutrients of flax, hemp, and similar oils are best reserved for cold preparations and use as supplements.

The Essential Nutrients

Our bodies are laboratories for nature, mixing and matching the foods we eat, separating them into fundamental compounds, and making new nutritional elements. These intermediate compounds are the metabolites forming the bridge between our meal and their destination in the physical body. Our digestive process makes what it needs from the foods we eat, breaking nutrients apart, reassembling them, and creating the intermediate metabolites. From these, tissues are built, organs function, and the immune system oversees it all.

Most nutrients consumed in foods can be refigured by the digestive process into metabolites the body needs. There are some, however, that are catalysts that cannot be created by other nutrients. These are the **essential nutrients** and need to be consumed in the diet. The essential nutrients, of which there are about fifty, are cofactors for the production of necessary metabolic compounds. Included are proteins, eight amino acids, vitamins, minerals, two fatty acids, water, oxygen, and light. These are the known factors, with new compounds discovered in ongoing research.

Vitamins, for example, were discovered by their absence. Scurvy and rickets were diseases relatively easily corrected by vitamin C and D once the compounds, or the foods containing them, were identified. Once the nutrient is supplied, the condition resolves if not of too long standing. As fundamental building blocks of all other compounds, essential nutrients are the catalysts and cofactors, raw materials for building the body and maintaining health. If not consumed as part of the diet in proper proportions, disease and degenerative conditions set in.

The **two *essential* fatty acids,** *alpha-Linolenic (LNA) acid* and *linoleic acid (LA),* build all the lipid compounds the body needs. They are best consumed in close to equal proportions, as they play different and contrasting roles in the body. They are equally necessary and vital for health. Their importance when first isolated caused them to be given a vitamin name, *Vitamin F factor.* The vitamin name is seldom used today, when the popular preference is for *essential fatty acid,* or *EFA.* Both essential fatty acids are polyunsaturated and their affinity for oxygen gives them an essential vitamin-like quality.

Alpha-linolenic acid (LNA), of the omega-3 family, is a super-unsaturated fatty acid with three double bonds (=) and can take up oxygen in multiple places. It's found in abundance in some fish oils, wild salmon, mackerel, and sardines, while important botanical sources are the seed oils like flax, hemp, perilla, chia, and walnut. Difficult to store, LNA's reactivity to oxygen can seriously cut into the shelf life of products containing it, unless protected by antioxidants.

Linoleic acid (LA), of the omega-6 family, and with two double bonds (=), has fewer places that attract oxygen than alpha-Linolenic acid and is somewhat more stable. With its greater stability, it is preferred by food manufactures and Big Agriculture. Linoleic acid can be found in the seed oils like safflower, sunflower, and grape-seed, and is significantly more available in the modern western diet than alpha-Linolenic acid, something that can be a problem for our health.

Essential Fatty Acids and Health

Part of what makes the essential fatty acids alpha-Linolenic (LNA) acid and linoleic acid (LA) so valuable is their chemical reactivity. The instability that ends in oxidation and rancidity in oils has the physiological benefit of carrying oxygen into and throughout the body. Absorbing sunlight, the EFAs increase the metabolic rate by carrying oxygen to provide fuel for the body. Oxidation is a life process needed for a healthy functioning organism.

The production of prostaglandins is another important function of the essential fatty acids. Prostaglandins are vital lipid compounds made by enzymatic actions on fatty acids. Produced throughout the body, they act as messenger molecules, controlling actions such as smooth muscle contraction and relaxation. Unlike hormones, which are produced in individual glands and travel through the body, prostaglandins are made where they are to be used. Adequate levels of EFAs in the diet insure that the prostaglandins are produced and function in the vicinity of where they are needed.

The body's inflammation response process is a valuable lesson in how the two essential fatty acids complement each other. When supplied in roughly equal amounts, the two essential fatty acids balance each other. The role they play in inflammation illustrates how they counterbalance each other in a healthy body.

The inflammatory response is a necessary action against microbial invasion or traumatic injury. Linoleic fatty acid stimulates inflammation, activating the healing process in the body. This natural response to warding off disease or healing from accidents maintains our health under a variety of circumstances. In contrast, the omega-3 alpha-Linolenic acid reduces inflammation and keeps it in check. When not required to repair a wound or fight invasion, inflammation is calmed and cells return to normal, ready to intervene again when necessary. By controlling inflammation, the body's response to pain and swelling are eased.

When inflammation is not caused by disease or trauma, but an imbalance of nutrients in food, the inflammatory state becomes chronic. Unless used to repair the body or overcome disease, inflammation can lead to degenerative states as tissues are chronically over-stimulated and inflamed. Over-consumption of linoleic acid fans inflammation, leading to chronic inflammatory conditions when left unchecked.

The maintenance of health depends on consumption of the two essential fatty acids. The proportional ratios balance the inflammation response, activating it in the event of injury or calming it during normal conditions. Ratios of omega 6 to 3 should be no greater than 6:1, with ratios of 3:1 to 1:1 closer to the ideal for health. Ratios have been as extreme as twenty omega 6 to one omega 3, 20:1, in the modern western diet. (Erasmus, p. 52.)

In addition to managing the inflammation response, essential fatty acids have a number of other benefits for the body. As primary constituents of cell membranes, they hold a light negative charge, enabling tissues to remain fluid and flexible, able to resist aggregating and clumping. EFAs regulate cell division and structure by assisting the flow of substances in and out of the cell walls. Cellular pressure and fluid balance within the cell structure is maintained.

Essential fatty acids help produce steroids and hormones, regulate nerve transmission, and act as the primary energy source for the heart muscle. Deficiencies and imbalances of the essential fatty acids play a significant role in the development of degenerative diseases such as heart disease, cancer, strokes, autoimmune diseases, and skin conditions. Vitally important for health, they affect growth, mental state, and vitality.

As transport mechanisms, essential fatty acids carry energy from sunlight throughout the body, absorbing oxygen to provide fuel for cells to function normally. The oxygen carried into the body binds with toxins and other unwanted elements, ushering them out of the body. As the main structural component of the body's cell membranes, including the skin, essential fatty acids convert nutrients into usable energy, making it available to the cells and tissues. Applied topically, the skin benefits from EFAs transporting nutrients into the body.

All fatty acids act as emollients on the skin, and the two essential fatty acids provide the greatest degree of emolliency. As the primary constituent of cell membranes, essential fatty acids support the health of skin tissues and its cellular structure. The combination of oil and water elements in moisturizers serves to soften and protect the outer skin layers. By helping to reduce moisture loss from the cells, essential fatty acids help the skin remain hydrated and pliable.

Important but Not "Essential"

Remember, the word "essential" applies to nutrients that synthesize compounds necessary for health and must be consumed in food. In the process, metabolites, small molecules that act as stepping stones to achieving the range of functions the body needs, are created. Linoleic and alpha-Linolenic acids are essential precursors of other vitally important fatty acids. These second stage fatty acids are vital too, and are sometimes helpful when added to the diet.

Eicosapentaenoic acid (EPA), *docosapentaenoic acid* (DHA), and *gamma-linolenic acid* (GLA) are vitally important fatty acids needed by the body and made from the two essential FAs, LA and LNA. Our bodies sometimes suffer inefficiencies converting from one necessary molecule to another, whether due to age, deficiencies, or disease. Obtaining necessary nutrients directly from their richest sources can help alleviate health problems. EPA and DHA are primarily found in marine foods, while GLA is found in plant oils, such as evening primrose, black currant, and borage seed.

GLA, a necessary part of the production of prostaglandins and proper functioning of the body, is converted from dietary linoleic acid when conditions are optimum. The consumption of GLA-rich oils can help improve health, bypassing the need for its production in the body. GLA and LNA fatty acids are almost identical forms, with one double bond difference. Even with this similarity, their actions and benefits vary and both are necessary for optimum health.

Medium-Chain Fatty Acids

Of the fatty acids, medium-chain saturated fatty acids (MCSFAs) have a unique and vital role to play in our health. These are the fatty acid chains that are eight, ten, and twelve carbons long. They are uniquely digestible and able to defend against microbial invasion. Found in abundance in coconut oil, other tropical oils, and in breast milk, they possess unusual and beneficial compounds and actions for the body.

As fatty acids with twelve carbon atoms or less, they behave differently in the digestive process than long chain fatty acids. When metabolized in the stomach into monoglycerides and free fatty acids, MCSFAs pass directly into the body to be used as a source of fuel. As relatively small molecules, the metabolic burden on the body's digestive process is reduced. Offering quick nourishment for the cells, they bypass the need for pancreatic enzymes and bile from the gallbladder. By not requiring energy for absorption, storage, or use, medium-chain saturated fatty acids stimulate metabolism and improve health (Fife, *Coconut Cures*, p.30–32).

Longer-chained fatty acids, fourteen carbons and above, do need digestive enzymes from the pancreas and bile from the gallbladder to be metabolized. They are stored as fat until the body needs them for energy.

Most unusual however, are the antimicrobial properties of these fatty acids. The MCSFAs are lauric acid, caprylic acid, and capric acid, which are C12:0, C10:0, and C8:0 respectively. They possess the uncommon ability to fight infectious and parasitic conditions in the body. The digestive process breaks down the triglycerides into fatty acids and a glycerol molecule, a monoglyceride, and free fatty acids. The now-free fatty acids create compounds unique and specialized in their ability to fight invading organisms that would harm health.

The monoglycerides formed from the medium-chain fatty acids are monolaurin, from lauric acid, monocaprylin from caprylic acid, and monocaprin from capric acid. The nature of these compounds is to act against viruses, bacteria, and protozoa by destroying the fatty coatings on the cell walls of the invading organisms. After being weakened, the body's own defenses are able to breach the vulnerable cell walls of the invaders and remove them. It is this protective ability of the MCT (medium-chained triglycerides) in breast milk that protects the newborn infant while his or her immune system develops (Fife, *Coconut Cures*, p. 32, 45–46).

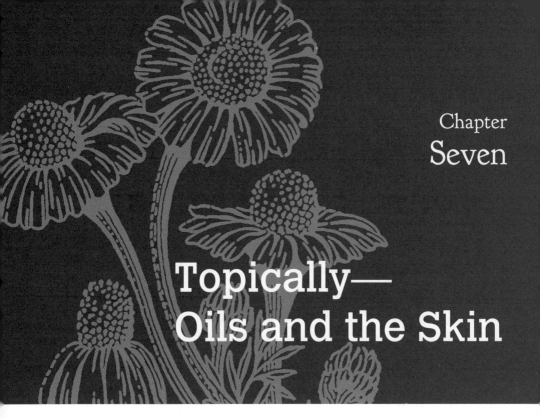

Chapter
Seven

Topically—
Oils and the Skin

Emollients, humectants, and occlusive agents are terms closely associated with skin care. **Emollient**, from the Latin *emollire,* means "to soften." This is a term that can be applied to all oils, as they improve the feel and appearance of the skin by overcoming dryness and protecting against water loss. An emollient creates a light barrier on the skin surface.

Humectant, from the Latin *humectus,* moist, or from *humere,* to be moist. A humectant is a substance that draws water to itself. Glycerin, the back bone or the "palm" of the triglyceride, is a humectant drawing water to itself from the environment. Glycerin can also draw moisture from lower layers of skin to the surface, and under adverse conditions dry it out. Newer humectants are made from honey, while others are manufactured synthetically. Propylene glycol is a synthetic humectant.

Occlusive agents, from "occlude," or in Latin, *occlusus,* create a physical barrier on the skin to keep moisture in the skin layers and prevent it from escaping. The long-chain saturated fatty acids like stearic and palmitic acids, and the waxes, are occlusive agents. Petroleum jelly is a synthetic occlusive agent.

The Skin Is an Organ

As the largest organ of the body, the skin is made up of three general layers: the epidermis, the dermis, and the subcutaneous layer. Each layer performs a myriad of functions maintaining and protecting the body as a whole and producing necessary compounds like vitamin D.

The outermost layer, the epidermis, is in turn made up of five layers, the outermost of which is called the **stratum corneum**, meaning *horned layer* in Latin. Once thought of as inert, a protective but inactive film, the stratum corneum is now recognized as biologically and chemically active. It performs two vital functions, **barrier function** (*protection*) and **passage function** (*movement*). Both are important tasks for the body as a whole. The degree to which these processes are healthy and perform normally determines the overall health of the skin.

The primary function of the stratum corneum is protection, preventing elements of the environment such as liquids, gases, objects, and unfriendly organisms from penetrating the skin. Internal functions are protected and the body held together as a unit; thus the *barrier function* is one of protecting our bodily integrity. The stratum corneum also functions as a permeable membrane, allowing a two-way *passage* into and out of the body. The passage function moves moisture in the form of perspiration, along with toxins and waste, out of the skin layers. From the outside in, skin absorbs moisture, oxygen, light, and nutrients, including fatty acids, moving them inwards to the body. Light passing into the lower skin layers also makes vitamin D, which is one of the passage function's especially vital roles.

Cerimides, a mix of lipids and skin cells with waxes, cholesterol, and free fatty acids, form the outermost layer, the stratum corneum. These lipids fill the space between *corneocytes,* cells no longer living, to protect the underlying tissues against dehydration, chemicals, infection, and mechanical wear and tear. Fatty acids produced in the skin layers and those obtained in natural oils play a large part in maintaining skin health. Lipids in the skin are vital to preserving moisture in cell membranes. They maintain suppleness and tone by preventing water from escaping, while also protecting skin cells from environmental stresses.

Stratum corneum lipids & corneocytes	
Cerimides, waxes	50%
Cholesterol	25%
Free fatty acids	10%
Corneocytes	remainder

The way these lipids are combined and organized determines the health of the stratum corneum and the skin as a whole. When functioning properly, a protective and permeable membrane performs multiple operations. When impaired, the function of the outermost layers fails, and skin conditions like eczema and dermatitis result. When compromised by allergens and pathogens, the skin barrier becomes inflamed, irritated, red, and skin diseases can result. Maintaining the stratum corneum is central to skin health.

Collagen, another vitally important part of the skin structure, is a protein complex of amino acids that represents nearly a third of the proteins in the body. Found in tendons, ligaments, bone, and skin, collagen is tough and strong, and makes up the connective tissue and protein cement that holds the body tissues together. Collagen functions in the skin to keep the tissues supple, firm, and elastic, and its loss leads to wrinkling and sagging tissues. Anti-aging treatments emphasize collagen support and replenishment for this reason.

Fatty Acids, Sebum, and the Skin

Fatty acids are ubiquitous in nature. Found in all living forms, plant and animal alike, they enable life processes to unfold throughout the life span of the organism. With plant oils and skin producing and sharing many of the same fatty acids, there is great compatibility. A proper balance of oils helps protect and repair tissues, but deficiencies of essential fatty acids can result in a variety of skin conditions and problems.

Skin produces its own fatty acids, making up 90% of the sebaceous lipids on the skin surface. Called **sebum** and produced in the sebaceous glands, these lipids are necessary for keeping the skin and hair supple and pliable. Attached to hair follicles, sebaceous glands produce the fatty acids that maintain the integrity and health of the skin. Of particular importance in addition to maintaining suppleness, sebum acts as the skin's innate immune system and operates as an immune organ. Able to produce antimicrobial compounds and perform pro- and anti-inflammatory functions, it controls wound healing and transports vitamins and antioxidants to the skin's inner and surface layers.

Integral to the optimum functioning of the skin, sebaceous glands are located over most of the body, with concentrations on the face, head, chest, and upper back. The sebum, or skin lipids, is called the "acid mantle" and can ward off bacterial infection, protecting all the layers. Fatty acids, which by nature are slightly acidic, create a surface environment inhospitable to microorganisms and bacteria. As the lipid cocktail of the stratum corneum, sebum provides a protective barrier, maintaining health and enabling the lower skin layers to function normally. Sebum is a complex mixture of triglycerides, waxes, free fatty acids, squalene, and cholesterol.

Sebum lipids	
Triglycerides	41%
Waxes, monoesters	25%
Free fatty acids	16%
Squalene	12%
Cholesterol	3%

The sebum also produces a uniquely human fatty acid, sapienic acid, C16:1, named from *Homo sapiens*. Formed by enzymatic action in the skin's sebaceous glands, it is a major portion of sebum. Enzymes acting on saturated palmitic acids, C16:0, make sapienic acid, a secondary fatty acid metabolite. As an isomer of palmitoleic acid, C16:1, sapienic acid differs only in its omega classification, which is omega-10. Sapienic acid converts to sabaleic acid, C18:2, a two-carbon extension. These uniquely human fatty acids perform a number of functions, including preservation of cellular health, regulating hormones, and other physiologic processes. The skin's own lipids combined with plant oils complement each other, providing active and passive smoothing, soothing, and protective effects.

Allergens, or Everyone Is Allergic to Something

Allergens are substances that produce sensitivities in some people but are not toxic to the population as a whole. All substances, including oils, can potentially possess allergenic properties. A friend with a severe celiac condition can barely stand to look at my bottle of oat seed oil, never mind removing the lid and smelling or handling it. She had no desire to experiment on any level. Wheat germ oil could also be an allergen for a person with such a condition.

Nuts are allergens to many people and the oils can be as well. Peanut, primarily, but also almond, hazelnut, pecan, brazil nut, and others can cause mild to serious reactions in those who are sensitive. Mangos, from the same botanical family as poison oak, are allergens for some people. In addition, allergenic properties can be present across a species. The butter from mango seeds can cause sensitivities for those with a mango allergy, as can marula and pistachio oils, which share the same botanical family. Rubber trees and shea trees share a similar botanical family, and individuals who are allergic to latex can also be sensitive to shea butter as well.

The importance of labeling all ingredients cannot be overstated. That keeps the public informed of possible complications to themselves, friends, or family members. However, people can also react to an ingredient or combination without knowing they are in fact allergic. If an allergen is known, it can be avoided with proper labeling, but sensitivities do occur where they haven't manifested in the past. Modifying recipes is not difficult and can be done by substituting similar ingredients, like a seed oil for a nut oil. No one product or combination will work for everyone, but with awareness of the problem, something can be found to work for most everyone.

Oils and Problems of Skin Health

Healthy skin depends on the integrity and balance of the stratum corneum. Skin conditions, including acne, occur when the ratios of lipids and fatty acids are out of balance. All living organisms and systems strive to maintain homeostasis, a dynamic balance within natural functions. Deficiencies of any of the essential nutrients throw off this balance and eventually manifest as disease.

Those with skin problems often have a damaged permeability layer that corresponds to low linoleic acid levels. This fatty acid makes up 14% of the ceramides, the waxes that constitute 50% of the stratum corneum, an important component of the barrier function. Deficiencies of linoleic fatty acid lead to dry scaly skin and hair, and slow-healing wounds.

Acne, it appears, is a result of an under-supply of linoleic acid, while monounsaturated palmitoleic and the human sapienic acids are over-produced by as much as 60%. Excess sebum builds in the tissues, causing the glands and hair follicles to become clogged. With the pores blocked, the condition becomes chronic and ultimately inflamed. Scaling, dryness, and skin problems are often caused by linoleic acid deficiencies, which can be made worse by excessive intake or use of oleic and other monounsaturated fatty acids. The skin's problems are exacerbated by increased sebum production when it is least wanted or needed.

The barrier function of the skin, in particular, needs linoleic acid in sufficient quantities to maintain and repair it. In studies, linoleic acid made available to the skin in the diet and topically has restored the barrier function in as little as a month. An understandable and common reaction to help alleviate the condition of excess oil is avoidance of all oils on the skin, but it is treatment *with* oils that can return the skin to normal. Recommended treatments often banish any and all oils in an attempt to actively dry the skin of excess oils and sebum. A better approach is to provide the missing fatty acids.

Saturated palmitic fatty acid, along with linoleic acid, can help calm the skin and return it to balance. Improved diet and essential fatty acid supplementation is also recommended to provide the necessary nourishment for regaining a healthy balance. Minimal use of monounsaturated fatty acids, including oleic acid, is recommended until the skin's health and balance is restored. Oleic acid in healthy balanced skin is beneficial, but it does not replace a deficiency of other fatty acids, especially an essential one.

Treating problem skin with combinations of fatty acids requires choosing the best oil or oils to supply the skin with what it is missing. Oils generally have dominant, secondary, and lesser fatty acid structures. The feel and function of fatty acids on the skin varies depending on saturation, carbon chain length and mix of all the fatty acids contained in a particular oil. Fatty acid tables identify the composition of oils and can help with choosing oils appropriate for the condition.

Oils and Skin Aging

It is a fact of life that we age, and along with the rest of the body, our skin changes over time. Many billions of dollars (as well as other currencies) have been spent trying to slow the process, even attempting reversal of the inevitable. This is not healthy or realistic. Caring for the skin with natural, non-processed foods in a diet high in vegetables and quality fats, drinking lots of clean water, and avoiding synthetic chemicals in skin care products is the best anti-aging beauty treatment for the skin.

Oils used in the diet and directly on the skin can mitigate the aging process considerably. What oils are used and when is a major theme of this book. **For cooking,** saturated butter, ghee, coconut, and palm oils are preferred, as they don't break down in the presence of heat. The omega-9 oils like olive, sesame, and macadamia can be used for light cooking, warming, and for dressing salads and dipping. The omega-6 polyunsaturated oils, like grape-seed, evening primrose, and corn, will oxidize with high heat, so they should only be used for dressings, dipping and supplements. The omega-3 flax, hemp, and chia seed oils should never be heated and should be stored in the refrigerator. Use them as supplements and in cold dishes to keep the oils fresh.

A feared sign of skin aging is the appearance of dark **skin spots** on the backs of the hands, arms, and face. These spots, which are not natural freckles, come from consuming unstable oils and are a type of oxidation.

Cooking with saturated oils that are stable when heated, rather than the polyunsaturated oils, slows formation of the spots and causes existing ones to fade. Increasing consumption of plant-based antioxidants can also help mitigate unwanted oxidation. Colorful reds, oranges, greens, and yellows in foods is a sign of the presence of antioxidant compounds that protect skin and body. Oxygen, like the sun, is necessary for life, and guarding against damage is easier than correction.

Oils, Sun, and Tanning

Oils produced from trees grown in tropical areas contain a number of compounds that protect against damage from the sun's rays while allowing natural and vital vitamin D formation in the lower skin layers. Coconut oil, cocoa butter, shea butter, babassu, mango butter, and tamanu are a few of the tropical oils offering the best sun protection. The skin is provided with the raw materials necessary to protect itself against damage, while allowing light to perform the important function of making vitamin D in the skin.

A personal note on growing up in the tropics: in those far off days of the 1950s and 60s, tanning darkly was accepted. Our sunning oils were combinations of coconut oil and cocoa butter, not mineral oil or synthetic sunscreens. Now, living in the Pacific Northwest, I never use sunscreen, needing the Vitamin D that the occasional sun makes in my skin. If I lived in the southern desert, I would have to alter how I lived with the sun, avoiding the hot middle of the day and using the tropical oils for protection when outside in the sun.

The skin is a living organ, not an impermeable barrier. Synthetic chemicals in sunscreens and mineral oil can harm the skin in the presence of solar radiation. By having to overcome the effects of both the sun and incompatible and non-physiologic chemicals, the skin is overwhelmed and stressed, leading to damaged tissues. The antioxidant compounds in tropical butters support skin cell function with natural and nourishing sun protective elements.

In the West, we have been repeatedly warned to fear the sun, but without it, life on planet earth would cease to exist. Coming to terms with how to protect against damage while enhancing the benefits we get from the sun is the best form of skin care. A food and skin care diet that relies on high quality fats and oils provides the skin tissues the compounds needed to remain in good condition throughout the span of a lifetime.

Oils and Skin Care

Oils used on the face and body should be as natural and organic as possible. Simple oils can be used to cleanse the face of makeup and dirt, by applying oil to the skin and wiping away the excess with a cloth or tissue. A hot washcloth placed over oiled, clean skin hydrates and supplies the face with phytoelements contained in the oil. The lighter oils, such as the omega-6 and omega-3 oils, make wonderful facial oils, either singly or in combination. Some oils are high in vitamin C, others in carotenes and pro-vitamin A compounds, minerals, and antioxidants. Applying them directly to the skin makes these nutrients available to skin cells. We'll discuss the types and uses of the different oils in the section on working with oils.

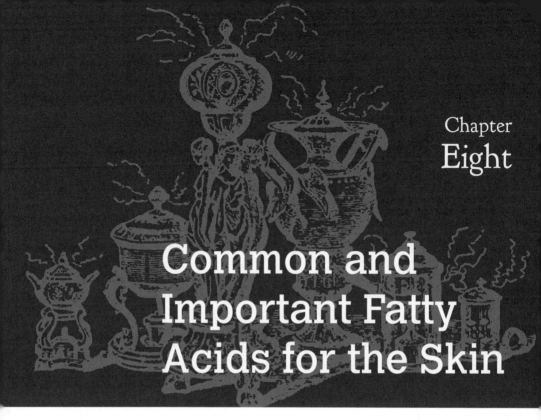

Common and Important Fatty Acids for the Skin

There are perhaps forty or fifty common fatty acids, and the number increases to over five hundred when rare, unique, and isomers of fatty acids are counted. For example, oleic acid is a very common fatty acid found in all oils, while ricinoleic acid is found in only one type of oil, castor oil. Lauric acid is found generously in a few oils, but in exceedingly small amounts in others. Erucic acid is found in significant percentages in mainly one botanical family, Brassica (the cabbage family). In this section, we'll look at the common fatty acids by type and how they affect the skin. We'll also review a few that stand out as unusual or unique to plant-based oils.

Essential and Polyunsaturated Fatty Acids

All fatty acids protect the skin, but the essential fatty acids (EFAs) are particularly important for its good health and normal functioning. Just as with the body as a whole, essential fatty acids have important roles to play for healthy skin. These are optimally supplied in the diet by food or supplementation, but can also be used externally. Oils high in these important fatty acids, like rosehip seed and black currant, have a particular nutty scent that some people love, while others don't. The scent can be modified by mixing with other oils and essential oils. The reactivity of polyunsaturated fatty acids with oxygen needs to be addressed in the making of products, or shelf life can be disappointingly short. Antioxidants like vitamin E are often added to prolong shelf life.

The omega-6 **linoleic acid,** LA, C18:2, is a particularly important fatty acid for skin health. The barrier and passage functions of the skin must be optimal, able to absorb or repel according to environmental conditions or current skin needs. Harmful bacteria, chemicals, and plain old dirt are kept out when these functions are working properly, while moisture and nutrients, including fatty acids, are absorbed into the skin layers. Linoleic acid plays a crucial role in maintaining the barrier and passage functions.

Oils high in linoleic acid absorb quickly and deeply into the skin layers. The quick absorption carries additional plant nutrients into the deeper layers of the skin to nourish and condition the cells. Grape-seed, safflower, evening primrose, and passion fruit seed oils are high in linoleic acid.

The other essential fatty acid, omega-3 **alpha-Linolenic acid,** LNA, C18:3, is particularly vital to the health of the skin and body. LNA is converted to EPA (eicosapentaenoic acid) and DHA (ocosahexaenoic acid), two fatty acids also found in fish oils. Anti-inflammatory and internally protective of the circulatory system, these acids perform functions particularly important for healthy skin.

As the essential fatty acid responsible for curbing inflammation, LNA helps to relieve itching, redness, and irritation of the skin. Protective, nourishing, and very light, oils with high ratios of both essential fatty acids, LNA and

LA, absorb incredibly quickly and easily. Produced primarily in seeds, high percentages of LNA are found in red raspberry, walnut, blackberry, chia, and flax seed oils.

Gamma-Linolenic acid, GLA, C18:3, an omega-6 fatty acid, is not an essential fatty acid, as it can be made from linoleic acid, but plays an important part in maintaining the health of the skin and body. Anti-inflammatory and immune supporting properties soothe redness, irritation, and itching. Wounds are healed and scarring minimized by nutrients necessary for regenerating skin cells.

Difficult skin conditions such as psoriasis, eczema, and dermatitis have been improved or corrected in studies with the use of GLA in the diet. Animal studies report that GLA slows excessive and pathological growth of skin cells, the characteristic of psoriasis. This study was conducted with oral doses of GLA-containing oil, but topical applications would help as well. Gamma-Linolenic acid is also beneficial for aging skin, as it helps maintain moisture levels and supports the skin's barrier function. As an omega-6 fatty acid, the oils high in GLA absorb quickly and deeply, leaving no oily residue on the surface of the skin. Borage, evening primrose, and black currant seed are the oils with significant percentages of GLA.

Monounsaturated Fatty Acids

Monounsaturated fatty acids are some of the most common found in nature, in plant and animal species alike. They are relatively stable against oxidation and hold up well in warmer climates. Produced by our own sebum, oleic and palmitoleic acids, as well as the human fatty acid sapienic acid, are all monounsaturates.

Oleic acid, C18:1, is an omega-9 fatty acid, its name derived from the olive. Making up 30% of the natural fatty acids of the skin, it is by far the most common fatty acid found in vegetable oils. It is also a significant part of animal fats, along with solid saturated fatty acids. Olive and avocado oils are good sources of oleic acid, with macadamia, camellia, and hazelnut oils also often containing higher percentages, up to 80%.

On the skin, oleic acid helps maintain suppleness, flexibility, and softness. Highly compatible with the sebum, the lipids of the stratum corneum remain semi-fluid, able to carry nutrients deeply into the skin layers. Oleic acid moisturizes by creating a fine protective film of nourishing monounsaturated fatty acids on the skin. Anti-inflammatory and regenerative properties maintain skin health, and the fatty acid is utilized and absorbed well. As a commonly available fatty acid, all oils contain some oleic acid, even if in small amounts. Its affinity with healthy skin function makes oleic acid a staple of good skin care.

When linoleic acid is deficient in the skin, oleic acid and other monounsaturated fatty acids can make problem skin worse by increasing sebum production. Minimal use of monounsaturated fatty acids, including oleic acid, is recommended until the skin's health is restored. Oleic acid is beneficial for healthy balanced skin but not necessarily for one that is deficient in an essential fatty acid.

Palmitoleic acid, C16:1, an omega-7 monounsaturated fatty acid, was discovered in palm oil, thus the *palm* of its name. Similar to saturated palmitic acid, it also contains a sixteen-carbon chain, but is monounsaturated with one double bond. Found in all tissues, palmitoleic acid is an important part of skin lipids. Produced by the sebaceous glands, it forms about 20% of sebum and protects against infectious agents. Palmitoleic acid is an isomer of the skin's own sapienic acid, also C16:1, and provides similar protective and antimicrobial actions for maintenance of healthy skin functions. (Remember, isomer is the term for two molecules with the same chemical formula but a different arrangement of atoms. The compounds are very similar but not identical.)

The production of palmitoleic acid in the skin decreases with age, so it's an excellent fatty acid supplement for mature skin care. As an anti-microbial, palmitoleic acid guards against infection, prevents damage from scratches, wounds, and burns, and stimulates the healing process. The fatty acid also maintains health in the mucus membranes, and is able to protect the skin from sun damage. Palmitoleic acid is a beneficial fatty acid present in very small amounts in many oils, but is generously supplied in a few: macadamia nut, sea buckthorn fruit, and Chilean hazelnut oils, in the amounts of 20%, 34%, and 25% respectively.

Saturated Fatty Acids

Saturated fatty acids function as barrier lipids. They are occlusive and protective, coating the skin and absorbing slowly, if at all. Not readily or deeply taken up by the tissues, they are excellent for protection against harsh elements, wind, cold, sun, and dryness. They are compatible with skin lipids, and preferable to petroleum oils and jellies for barrier protection. Being saturated, these oils have no omega designation, as they have no double bonds.

Stearic acid, C18:0, a long-chain saturated fatty acid with 18 carbon molecules, is used to harden soaps and emulsify products. It is waxy, solid, and has a relatively high melting point, and by itself is a hard wax suitable for candles. As a component of many oils, it provides stiffness in butters and thickness in unsaturated oils. Animal fat contains a large percentage of stearic acid, and is the usual source of the raw material.

Sebum is made up of about 11% stearic acid. As a saturated fatty acid, stearic acid helps support and protect the barrier function of the skin. Found in saturated vegetable butters and oils and animal fats, accompanied by other naturally occurring saturated and unsaturated fatty acids, stearic acid is a plus in protective care of the skin.

Palmitic acid, C16:0, a long-chain saturated fatty acid, makes up about 22% of sebum. Found in high percentages in vegetable butters and the heavier oils, it is one of the most common fatty acids in nature. It is another fatty acid derived from the palm, where it was first discovered. As a saturated fatty acid it remains stable and does not oxidize. Along with cholesterol and ceramides, palmitic acid has some antimicrobial properties, which protect the skin from unwanted penetration of environmental substances. It is also said to cause cancerous cells to self-destruct, and studies have observed it retarding cell proliferation. As a saturated fatty acid it helps form an occlusive layer, protecting the barrier function of the skin.

Myristic acid, C14:0, a saturated fatty acid with a chain of four fewer carbon atoms than stearic acid, is able to penetrate the skin. Myristic acid, along with myristoleic acid, C14:1, were both originally identified in and named for *Myristica fragrans* the botanical name of the nutmeg tree. As one of the fatty acids found in the highly valued sperm whale oil popular in the nineteenth and early twentieth centuries, myristic acid is sought-after for skin care.

Myristic acid is present in a number of vegetable oils and butters in small quantities, and makes up part of the skin lipids or sebum. Due to its relatively short carbon chain, myristic acid provides a light protective barrier of a saturated fatty acid. Closer to lauric acid (12:0) than stearic (18:0) in action, it is fairly easily absorbed. Myristic acid is also anti-inflammatory and able to regenerate and repair the skin barrier function. It forms 15% of palm kernel oil, 2.5% of tamanu oil, and 2% of palm oil, while it is generally less than one percent in a number of other oils.

Lauric acid, C12:0, is a medium-chained fatty acid whose impact on health has been discussed in the previous section on medium-chained saturated fatty acids. Although saturated, its medium-length chains of only 12 carbon atoms allow easy absorption by the skin externally and internally. Lauric acid is one of the free fatty acids found in sebum, making it highly compatible with normal skin functions. Its conversion to monolaurin promotes antimicrobial activity against bacteria and viruses in the skin layers. Coconut, palm kernel, babassu butter, and other tropical oils are high in lauric acid. Temperate climate oils produce only very small or trace amounts of the fatty acid.

Very-Long-Chain Fatty Acids

The very-long-chain fatty acids have chains of 20 carbons and above. They are not nearly as prevalent in nature as the long chains of 14 to 18 carbon atoms, but play an important role in lipid balance. In the skin, they make up a very small percentage of the fatty acids, but are vital for its health and balance. It could be said that they perform as necessary *trace fatty acids*, in the same way as trace minerals. Oils high in the very-long-chain fatty acids are unusually stable, resisting oxidation that readily occurs in shorter-chain unsaturated fatty acids.

Gadoleic acid, also called **eicosenoic acid**, C20:1, is a very-long-chain omega-9 monounsaturated fatty acid first found in cod liver oil. Present in small amounts in many vegetable oils, and in large quantities in a few, the long chains provide properties that protect the barrier function of the skin. Jojoba oil contains between 50 to 80% gadoleic acid, and meadowfoam oil contains 60%. The long chains contribute stable properties to oils, protecting the skin's outer layers from damage by oxidation.

Erucic, or **docosenoic acid**, C22:1, another omega-9 fatty acid, has a chain of 22 carbon atoms and is monounsaturated. Found in small quantities in a wide range of oils, it plays a large part in the cabbage, or *Brassica* family: abyssinian oil contains 60%, broccoli seed oil 49%, and daikon radish seed oil has 34%. Canola or rapeseed oil has had the erucic fatty acid bred out of the seed, while in camelina oil, another cabbage family member, the fatty acid content is naturally a smaller 2%. Meadowfoam seed oil is an exception: although it is not a member of the cabbage family, it has 12% erucic acid.

In the mid-1970s, Canada and the US limited erucic acid to 5% or less in oils for human consumption. Studies done on rats to determine the safety of erucic acid were conducted and cited as the reason for the development of a low erucic acid oil, later named canola oil. Except it was later found that the heart damage thought to be caused by the erucic fatty acid in the rats was also caused by sunflower oil containing no erucic acid. Rat metabolism of oils is not the same as human metabolism, yet this poorly devised study created a large new industry. Rapeseed was bred for reduced erucic acid content in Canada, and now provides a low-erucic acid seed for oil production. Not all countries keep erucic acid-containing oils off the market, and Asian cultures commonly use high erucic acid oils like mustard and non-hybridized rape, containing up to 40% of the fatty acid. (Erasmus, p. 117.)

Erucic acid has the isomer brassidic acid, which is similar to, though not the same as, brassic acid C22:2, another fatty acid also from the cabbage family. Oils with significant percentages of these very-long-chain fatty acids feel wet but not oily, like a silicone. The action of erucic acid on the skin is primarily protective as a lipid layer and is stable against oxidation.

Erucic acid is also part of a combination known as "Lorenzo's oil," named for a child with a rare, inherited medical condition called adrenoleukodystrophy (ALD). The child was given two years to live by the medical establishment with no hope of cure. His parents began the search to help their son and after years of dedicated research, discovered what was to be named Lorenzo's oil, a combination of erucic acid and oleic acid, in a 4:1 mix, extracted from rapeseed oil and olive oil. Lorenzo was able to live into adulthood, dying 22 years after his original diagnosis, at the age of 30.

Behenic acid, C22:0, a fatty acid with a very long saturated chain, lends great stability to oils. The fatty acid was first discovered in moringa, an oil used in Egypt for thousands of years and found in Egyptian tombs. Moringa is known commercially as ben oil or behen oil because of its behenic acid content. Since its discovery, behenic acid has been found in praxci oil (from seeds of a South American tree) as well as peanut and rapeseed oils. Behenic acid is poorly absorbed by the body when eaten and causes cholesterol levels to rise. However, for topical use it is protective against oxidative damage, helping to keep products fresh for extended lengths of time. The moringa oil of the Egyptians is said to have had a shelf life of five years—long indeed for oil.

Unique and Uncommon Fatty Acids

Fatty acids can also be unique and unusual, represented only in single plant families or varieties. Having looked at the more common and important fatty acids, we'll now look at two unusual fatty acids found in castor and pomegranate seed oil, as well as the conjugated fatty acids.

Ricinoleic acid, C18:1, an omega-9 monounsaturated fatty acid, constitutes up to 90% of the fatty acids found in castor oil. This unusual fatty acid has pain-alleviating, anti-fungal, and anti-bacterial properties. Castor oil, used for its healing properties, has the ability to deeply penetrate the skin, and is a traditional home remedy for many conditions.

What is unusual about ricinoleic acid is the placement of a hydroxyl group (-OH) on the 12th carbon of an 18-carbon chain. The fatty acid is more polar than other 18-carbon fatty acids, and is more easily absorbed by the skin given its chain length.

Ricinoleic Acid

Castor oil can thicken and regenerate skin tissues, helping to preserve the integrity of mature and damaged complexions. A very viscous oil, thick and heavy, it is also easily absorbed. Once absorbed, it is taken up by the internal organs and stimulates fluid movement of lymph and blood in the body. As an humectant, it attracts moisture to it and thus to the skin.

Punicic acid, C18:3, is an omega-5 fatty acid found in large quantities in pomegranate seed oil (75%) as well as the seeds of snake and bitter gourd. Named from *Punica granatum,* the botanical name for pomegranate, punicic acid is a conjugated fatty acid, having both cis and trans configuration naturally. This form causes the carbon chains to be twisted, making pomegranate oil feel thick and heavy despite its unsaturated characteristics.

Punicic acid has unique properties that fight inflammation and regenerate tissues. The skin's natural functions are strengthened by the fatty acids' unique makeup. Punicic acid protects the internal moisture balance of the skin, while keeping unwanted environmental elements out. As skin matures and ages, normal physiologic functions slow. Punicic acid helps maintain healthy skin by supporting collagen production and protecting against environmental effects of sun and weather. Pomegranate seed oil, with its high percentage of punicic acid and plant nutrients, is valuable for mature skin care.

Conjugated fatty acids are of two broad types, with many isomers. What is most notable about them is their unusual carbon chains. Conjugated fatty acids consist of carbon chains that have alternating double bonds, in both trans and cis configurations naturally, which causes the strands to twist. Like we see in punicic acid in pomegranate seed oil, the trans and cis configurations cause the fatty acids to be thicker than if they were simply cis. The molecules won't lie down in a straight, flat line, which causes a feeling of thickness and heaviness in the oils. Health benefits are attributed to these types of natural fatty acids, including treating and preventing skin cancers, skin conditions, rejuvenating skin cells, and repairing the stratum corneum. They are very effective at reducing inflammation, improving skin tone, moisturizing cells, lightening skin, and enhancing skin elasticity.

The most common **conjugated fatty acid** is **(CLA) conjugated linoleic acid**, found generously in animal sources, particularly meat and dairy products. It is produced by the intestinal bacteria of grass-fed ruminants such as cows, goats, and sheep. A family of 28 isomers, conjugated linoleic acid has properties similar to linoleic acid; it is 18 carbons long with two double bonds, but is conjugated.

The closely related botanical representative of conjugated fatty acids is **conjugated linolenic acid (CLnA)**, which could be considered the omega 3 of the conjugated fatty acids. Only trace amounts of CLA is found in the seeds of plants. A CLnA with 18 carbons and three double bonds, punicic acid (C18:3), found in pomegranates, is the plant world's top source. Punicic acid is also found in snake gourd and bitter gourd seeds. Eleostearic acid (C18:3), found in pomegranate and cherry kernel oil, is also a conjugated CLnA. Calendic acid from pot marigold, calendula seeds, is another botanical source of CLnA, containing as much as 65% of the total fatty acids. Research is being done in Europe to develop calendula as an oil seed crop. To date, "calendula oil" has been made by macerating the flowers in a base oil. The pressed oil from the seeds will be a welcome addition for natural skin care.

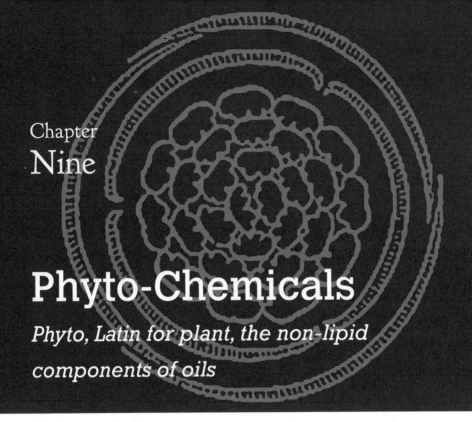

Phyto-Chemicals

Phyto, Latin for plant, the non-lipid

components of oils

Phyto-chemicals, the plant-produced compounds found in all of nature, number in the thousands and protect and prevent disease, serving the health of the plant. When we consume the plants and their oils, we benefit from these compounds as well. Antioxidants, vitamins, tannins, sterols, polyphenols, and terpenes are all phytochemicals that guard our health and nourish our bodies.

Oils consist primarily of fatty acid lipids, in quantities of 95 to 99%. The non-lipid percentage is the *healing fraction*, the *unsaponifiable* extras that give oil its personality and identity. Uniquely individual combinations of compounds determine what makes one oil red and another green, one nutty-smelling and another fruit-scented. Of thousands of known phyto-chemicals, plant oils contain vitally important compounds for health. Many of the protective roles these compounds perform for the plants are shared with us when we consume the plants as food.

Two major classes of phytochemicals contribute innumerable compounds that benefit both plants and humans. Polyphenolic compounds and terpenes are found in plant tissues, including the seeds, nuts, and kernels. Natural **phenolic compounds** are antioxidant-rich, with thousands of protective elements guarding against disease, free radical damage, and pests, all while providing the intense coloration of fruits, vegetables, leaves, and nuts. **Terpenes** and **terpenoids** are the building blocks and structure of the plant world, creating the scents, nutrition, vitamins, hormones, and coloration of plants.

Of the thousands of phyto- chemical compounds, many are associated with the botanical oils. These elements include vitamins, minerals, flavonoids, lipid structures, and other plant chemicals that impact and benefit the skin and body. Since many of these are identified in books and papers on the oils, the following section lists some of the more common and important ones along with their properties.

The Necessity of Oxygen and Antioxidants

We breathe in oxygen and exhale CO_2. Once in the body, oxygen fuels our cells and organs, creating physical energy and warmth. Like logs burning in the fireplace on cold winter days, oxygen is necessary for combustion. The energy released keeps you warm. Neither the fire at home nor our internal fires can burn without oxygen. The body's metabolism uses food as fuel that releases energy for life processes. A diet high in plant compounds, minerals, and vitamins keep this fire burning brightly without burning out of control.

As important as oxygen is for life, it has another side. Oxygen can also damage cells and life forms. Without good nutrition in the form of essential nutrients and a ready supply of plant-based food high in antioxidants, the fire can burn past the fireplace and set the whole house aflame. Fire that burns beyond its rightful boundaries breaks down tissues that it is supposed to build up. Antioxidants are the protective compounds that hold the balance between life and cellular breakdown.

Able to counter the destabilizing action of oxygen, antioxidants protect cells and molecules from oxidative damage. Similar to rust on steel or the browning of an apple, these chemical reactions take place when electrons jump from one state to another, producing free radicals and unstable electrons. In the process, free radicals can cascade out of control and cause cellular damage, even cell death.

Although the flesh of apples turns brown when exposed to oxygen in the air (a process known as oxidizing), a little lemon juice brushed on the cut flesh keeps it white and fresh-looking. Vitamin C, an antioxidant contained in the juice, is what protects against the browning of oxidation. Antioxidants are the rescuers. By allowing themselves to be oxidized in the place of our cells, or the apple's flesh, antioxidant plant compounds step in and stop the oxidative cascade by inserting electrons into unstable atoms. They arrest the chain reaction, removing or neutralizing free radical electrons. The antioxidant protection of cells is probably the most important role that plants play in our diet and our skin care.

Phenolic Compounds

Phenolic compounds account for 40% of the carbon in the biosphere and provide both the broad range of colors and an all-encompassing shield that protects the botanical world. **Polyphenols**, from *poly,* many, and *phenol,* a class of organic chemicals found in plants, guard against the oxidation process. They are the structural form of antioxidants found in the botanical world. *Oxygen radical absorption capacity*, or ORAC, is a shorthand method for describing a protective function by an element or group of elements found in plants. There are over four thousand ORAC compounds in the plant kingdom, all of which protect the tissues and plant functions against free radical damage. When we use oils that possess compounds with high ORAC values in food or on our skin, they also protect our health from oxidative damage.

Polyphenols function in their parent plants by also defending against herbivores, UV radiation, wounding, environmental stresses, encroachment by other plants, invasive pathogens, pests, and fungi. Quinones, phenols, tannins, flavonols, isoflavones, furocoumarins, stilbenes, and hydrocinnamic acid are names of a few of these guardians. In addition to the elaborate and extensive protective blanket provided by the polyphenols, they also contribute the broad range of coloration in fruit, flower, roots, seeds, and nuts.

Polyphenols are under intense study for their disease-fighting potentials. Cancer research especially is focused on the many unique compounds that can combat or slow the progression of the disease. The fixed oils from plants and the compounds they contain are cited in numerous articles resulting from the research.

Polyphenols are present in all botanically based ingredients used in skin care, including the oils, hydrosols, butters, and essential oils. They are the compounds that are *essential* in essential oils. Polyphenols fall into two broad categories: flavonoids and non-flavonoid compounds.

Flavonoids

Flavonoids, derived from *flavus,* meaning yellow in Latin, are found throughout nature, with over 4,500 identified so far. Originally called vitamin P because of their important role in nutrition as a secondary metabolite, flavonoids' powerful anti-inflammatory, anti-microbial, and anti-allergic actions impact all layers of the skin. On the skin's surface, flavonoids protect the lipids of the stratum corneum. In the dermis, the middle skin layer where vitamin D is formed, flavonoids offer protection from free radical damage by UV rays. And in the hypodermis, the lowest skin layer, flavonoids protect the capillaries and blood flow that supply and feed the skin as a unit.

There are two types of flavonoids, **flavanols** with an *a* and **flavonols** with an *o*.

Flavanols

Catechins and **epicatechins**, types of flavonoids found in tea, berries, and dark-colored fruits and their oils, are a building block of tannins that help skin protect itself and heal. As powerful antioxidants, catechins help prevent damage from free radical activity while also providing antibiotic and antibacterial protection. Catechins also stimulate the production of naturally occurring protective enzymes, like glutathione, an enzyme produced by cells for use against toxins and free radicals. Being anti-inflammatory, they help reduce redness and irritations of the skin.

Proanthocyanidins, formed from catechins and epicatechins, are a form of flavanols with highly antioxidant properties. Said to be 200 times more powerful than vitamin C and 50 times more than vitamin E, they have a high ORAC value. When treated with an acid, they can break apart to become anthocyanins, creating the wide variety of fruit, flower, leaf, and root colors and the compound Cyanidin. Cyan is a green-blue color associated with nature's blues and purples.

Proanthocyanidins are sometimes referred to as *condensed tannins* and they account for astringency in a variety of plants. They play a role in stabilizing collagen and maintaining elastin, two critical proteins that make up connective tissues of the body including the skin. Found in grape seeds and grape skin, proanthocyanidins are also found in cranberry, black currant, green and black teas, and cocoa. With anti-mutagenic properties, they protect against damage to cells and unhealthy cell proliferation.

Flavonols, Flavones, and Isoflavones

Quercetin, from *Quercus*, the botanical name for oak, is a plant pigment flavonoid that gives many foods their color, including the reds in red onions and apples, as well as yellows, browns, and blues in other plants. Antiviral and anti-inflammatory, quercetin compounds maintain skin and body health. Antihistamine properties also protect against allergic reactions and irritations. Quercetin is also being studied for its ability to slow the progression of cancer cell growth.

Rutin, *quercetin rutinoside*, is a citrus flavonoid glycoside generously found in citrus family plants. Its name, however, is derived from the plant rue, *Ruta graveolens*. Rutin, a variation similar to the quercetin group, is a more powerful antioxidant and useful for UVA protection. Rutin also helps with circulation, and can be used topically to improve skin tone. Anti-inflammatory properties also help with histamine production, helping to control allergic reactions.

Non-Flavonoid Phenolic Acids

Phenolic acids, principally **gallic acid**, can take a variety of forms, whether as part of a tannin molecule or standing on its own. Antioxidant, anti-fungal, and antiviral, gallic acid is a protective compound found in many plants. Its astringent actions speed wound healing, and studies have shown that it can kill cancerous cells while preserving healthy cells. Found in pomegranate, witch hazel, evening primrose, mango butter, and tea, it is present in both oils and herbs.

Ellagic acid, with antioxidant, anti-bacterial, anti-inflammatory, antiviral, and antiseptic properties, protects skin collagen and promotes cellular regeneration. Ellagic acid's action helps thicken thin skin, improving its texture. Found in the oils of blackberry, pomegranates, raspberries, cranberries, walnuts, and pecans, the compound is a natural phenol that helps maintain the health of the skin. Another of the polyphenols under study in laboratory trials, it has shown the ability to slow cancer proliferation.

Tannins are astringent agents, possessing the same quality that causes the mouth to pucker when drinking tea or eating fruits such as quince or persimmons. Water-soluble, they act by binding tissues, beginning the body's healing process. By causing skin proteins to harden and dry, to pucker up and constrict, tissues are toughened and protected against external invasions. Tannins are what transforms animal hides into leather.

Tannins are also anti-viral, anti-inflammatory, and anti-bacterial, supporting tissue health and balance. Plant oils containing tannins create dry-feeling oils, with astringent properties able to help minimize pores and tighten tissues. Oils high in tannins include hazelnut, tea seed, or camellia, mango butter, grape-seed, rose hip seed, and jojoba. Used on the skin and in products, astringent oils feel less oily and absorb more readily than oils with low or no tannin content.

Malic acid, first found in apples, causes the sour, tart taste in fruits such as apples and berries, as well as in some vegetables. Associated with cell metabolism, it is an alpha-hydroxy acid and a stage of the citric acid cycle. The compound plays a role in energy production in the cells and acts as an energy source. The sour acids bind with toxic and unwanted metals, carrying them out of the body. In skin care, malic acid tightens pores, helping to smooth the skin of fine lines and wrinkles. A polyphenol antioxidant, malic acid is present in some nut and seed oils such as grape-seed, cranberry, and cucumber seeds and oil.

Hydroxycinnamates, the phenylpropanoids

Cinnamic acid, a powerful antioxidant with UV-protective properties, is found in shea and other tropical butters, cinnamon, and balsams like storax.

The acid compound penetrates the skin, helping to promote cell regeneration, a key property for its use in anti-aging treatments. By reducing the look of fine lines and wrinkles, skin is refreshed and tightened.

With a honey-like scent, cinnamic acid is also used in the perfume industry, and is a compound found in essential oils as well as fixed oils. Naturally occurring cinnamic acid found in the fixed oils is buffered by the fatty acids on the skin. Used as an isolated extract, cinnamic acid can have harmful side effects, including thinning skin, inability to retain moisture, and irritation. The compound acts as a precursor to other polyphenols, ferulic and caffeic acids.

Ferulic acid, a component of lignins and plant cell walls, is primarily found in cereals, especially the bran. A powerful antioxidant, ferulic acid possesses antibacterial properties, and reportedly shows promise fighting cancer by causing cancerous cells to self-destruct in its presence.

Extracts of ferulic acid are used in skin-lightening products. Melanin, the cellular pigment structure in the skin, dissipates the effect of the sun, by darkening the skin and making it less susceptible to damage from UVB rays. Ferulic acid acts to suppress melanin production by absorbing UV rays. By turning off the mechanism that activates melanin production, the skin is protected. As a bonus, ferulic acid's potency and ability to shield the skin is enhanced in the presence of ultra violet light.

Caffeic acid, found in cell walls of all plants, is another structural component of lignins and another powerful antioxidant able to outperform most others when tested. Despite the name, it is not related to caffeine. Caffeic acid protects cells against UV light exposure and free radical damage. It is also being studied for its cancer-fighting properties. Caffeic acid is particularly high in coconut oil, soy, and mango butter. In the body, caffeic acid can transform into ferulic acid, enhancing the properties that help protect the skin from the sun.

Rosmarinic acid is a form of caffeic acid ester found principally in the plants of the mint family *Lamiaceae,* which includes rosemary, lemon balm, sage, oregano, and perilla. Antioxidant and antimicrobial, it is used as a preservative in foods and skin care products. Its anti-inflammatory properties help to smooth the skin of fine lines while helping regenerate skin cells.

Lignans

Lignans are a polyphenol class of their own and able to transform into *phytoestrogens*, or plant estrogen. These are not to be confused with lignins with an *i*, which are structural functions of cells like bark and bran. Lignans, with an *a*, are metabolized in the digestive system by bacteria and protect the body by binding with estrogen receptors against excess or unhealthy estrogen. They act as antioxidants in and on the body, and are primarily found in seeds and other grains. Oats, flax, and sesame seeds are high in lignans. Consumed as a component of unrefined oils, they help to maintain hormone health and balance.

Terpenes and Terpenoids

Terpenes and terpenoids, compounds present in all living organisms, are some of the most wide-spread, naturally occurring elements of the plant world. They play vital roles in the physiology of plants and the cellular membrane. Chemical work on turpentine in the nineteenth century gave terpenes their name.

Both terpenes and terpenoids are present in all parts of the plant, and possess medicinal properties and biologic activity. Built from repeating isoprene units consisting of five hydrocarbons (C_5H_8), they are named according to the number of units: mono, di, or tri. Terpenes are highly aromatic, making up many of the compounds in essential oils.

Terpene	Isoprene Units	Carbon Atoms	Examples
Isoprene	1	5	basic isoprene unit of 5C
Monoterpenes	2	10	essential oils
Sesquiterpenes	3	15	essential oils
Diterpenes	4	20	resins, Vitamin A
Triterpenes	6	30	squalene, phytosterols
Carotenoids	8	40	vitamins, provitamin A

The difference between terpenes and terpenoids is the presence of oxygen in the latter and its absence in the former. A **terpene** is composed of carbon and hydrogen atoms, like our fatty acid chain minus its acid end, its oxygen. Vitamin A is a terpene; a diterpene, containing four isoprene units with 20 carbon atoms. **Terpenoids** are composed of carbon and hydrogen with the addition of oxygen. Our fatty acid chain, lipids, belong to the terpenoid group, as do the oil-soluble vitamins, saponins, carotenoids, essential oils, and phytosterols.

Phytosterols, from *phyto*, plant-derived sterol, are unsaturated solid alcohols of the steroid group, found in fatty tissues of plants and animals. Cholesterol is the only sterol produced by human and animal tissues in the liver, and is a main component of cell walls. Waxy in texture, cholesterol makes up much of our cellular walls along with the phospholipids. Cholesterol helps maintain cellular structure and health, as well as convert the sun's rays to vitamin D. *Ergosterol,* found in mushrooms, converts to vitamin D in the body through the action of the sun's rays. Both plant sterols and animal-produced cholesterol are vital for healthy cell functions.

Plant sterols are the botanical counterpart of cholesterol, and function in the body in similar ways. Generously supplied by the plant kingdom, there are over 200 phytosterols, found primarily in nuts, seeds, and whole grains. Common phytosterols include *beta-sitosterols, stigmasterols*, and *campesterols.* Found in vegetable oils, they figure prominently in skin care by calming inflammation, encouraging the formation of collagen, and protecting against its breakdown.

A study performed in Germany found that phytosterols in vegetable oils applied to the skin stimulate collagen formation. Collagen, the protein group that gives the skin its structure, breaks down as we age, causing the skin to wrinkle and thin. Using quality oils topically helps keep the skin collagen in good condition, slowing the effects of sun and time. By helping to decrease inflammation in skin tissues, phytosterols encourage elasticity, while protecting and repairing damage from excess UV rays of the sun.

Squalene, a natural thirty-carbon organic lipid compound, a triterpene, is produced by all plants and animals, including humans. Functioning in the synthesis of sterols, squalene is one of the most common lipids produced by human skin. Compatible with skin cells and absorbing quickly, squalene performs as an antioxidant, preventing age spots while protecting against sun damage. Its emollience helps the skin retain moisture, and antibacterial properties protect the skin while promoting healthy cellular growth. Studies on the nature of squalene have indicated that it may also fight the formation of cancerous cells. Squalene is often added to cosmetics and applied directly to the skin.

First found in shark liver oil, the most abundant source, squalene is also found in botanical sources, primarily olives, rice bran, and wheat germ, with lesser amounts in many other oils. Squalane, with an *a,* is the saturated form of squalene, and therefore more stable than the highly unsaturated squalene. Squalane is achieved by hydrogenation, and often found on ingredient labels. A new source of the compound, extracted from sugar cane, is commercially available as squalane. Both forms, squalene and squalane, are common additions to supplements, cosmetics, and skin care products.

Vitamins

Vitamins are vital nutrients that cannot be synthesized in the body. They belong to the *essential nutrient* category of compounds that must be consumed in the diet. Vitamins added to cosmetics as synthetic compounds or as plant extracts can help maintain skin health. Oil-soluble vitamins are stable elements and added to products in the oil phase. Water-soluble vitamin C presents problems of stability when added to products, as it oxidizes easily.

Carotenoids, the precursors of **vitamin A**, are terpenes consisting of eight isoprene units, and are exclusively found in botanical sources. Animals and humans cannot synthesize carotenoids and need to ingest them from plant-based foods. There are hundreds of carotenoid compounds in nature that are metabolized in the body, some of which convert to vitamin A. There are two forms of carotenoids, the *carotenes*, which often appear in the purple/red/orange color spectrum, and the *xanthophylls*, which have a yellow color that contributes to the green in leaves.

Carotenes, oil-soluble, oxygen-free molecules, protect and nourish the skin and body. Beta, alpha, gamma carotenes, and lycopene, are common forms. Color is a major distinguishing characteristic of the carotenes, ranging from violet to red to orange to yellow, although not all yellows are carotenes. Named from carrots, carotenes are found in carrot seed and root oils. Other deeply colored oils, such as the buriti palm, sea buckthorn berry, tomato seed, and carrot root oil, are extremely orange, even red-yellow in color. Used topically, they halt free radical damage in the tissues, protecting against damaging sun's rays.

The red-orange pigments aid the process of photosynthesis in plants by transmitting energy from light absorbed from chlorophyll. A naturally rich source of provitamin A, fifty of the known carotenoids are carotenes able to convert to retinol, an active form of Vitamin A.

Xanthophylls, water-soluble carotenoid molecules that contain oxygen, are found in leafy green plants like the kales, cabbage, and spinach. Xanthophylls include lutein and zeaxanthin. These carotenoids do not convert to vitamin A, but are powerful antioxidants in their own right.

Vitamin E is a family of related phenolic compounds that act as antioxidants. Grouped into three branches—tocopherols, tocotrienols, and the most recently isolated, tocomonoenol—they protect the cells of the body from oxidative stress. Donated hydrogen electrons from the hydroxyl (-OH) group cause free radicals to become nonreactive, stopping cascade reactions. Both tocopherol and tocotrienols occur in alpha, beta, gamma, and delta forms.

The *tocopherols group,* the most familiar form of Vitamin E, was first discovered in 1922. As a group, tocopherols are potent antioxidants, protecting tissues of the body from free radical damage and suppressing toxic peroxides generated by UV exposure on the skin. By reducing UV-caused toxicity, they protect cell membranes, reduce inflammation, and speed wound healing. Many vegetable oils produce tocopherols as natural protection against oxidation. Often added in storage, tocopherols slow oils from going rancid. Sesame, sunflower, olive, and walnut contain only tocopherols, but are absent the other forms of vitamin E.

Tocotrienols are not as well-known, but are more effective antioxidants—40 to 60 times more effective than the alpha-tocopherols. Structurally less saturated than the tocopherols, they are mobile and reactive. The smaller molecular size and greater mobility of tocotrienols increases their degree of absorption. Their potent anti-inflammatory properties protect skin against damage and stresses caused by a range of conditions. Found primarily in the cereal grains, such as rice bran, rye, barley, wheat germ, and oats, significant amounts of tocotrienols are also found in cranberry seed, blueberry seed, palm oils, and cocoa butter.

A new form of vitamin E, *tocomonoenol*, recently identified in palm oil, has significant radical scavenging properties similar to tocopherols. It is found in kiwi fruit peels and seeds and marine sources, with salmon eggs containing the highest concentrations. What was once simply called vitamin E has expanded into multiple branches. Sourcing raw materials as naturally as possible allows for the use of compounds that are not yet isolated, identified, or understood. Many vital contributions to our health have yet to be recognized and included.

Vitamin C, another vital nutrient for health, is a water-soluble compound and highly unstable. In the form of L-ascorbic acid, it oxidizes rapidly with oxygen when added to water. Skin care products containing unstable forms have little value if the vitamin oxidizes before use. Simple L-ascorbic acid will not hold in a formula containing water, oxidizing and turning yellow relatively quickly. Stable forms of the vitamin are available. Both an oil-soluble version, ascorbyl palmitate, or in compounds with minerals as magnesium ascorbyl phosphate (MAP), are photo and oxygen stable. Concentrated forms of vitamin C topically can cause irritation of the skin in some people, so should be used with caution.

Vitamin C benefits the skin in a number of ways, including the promotion of collagen production, repairing skin from conditions that cause wrinkling, dryness, and roughness, and supporting the skin's immune function. The best method of delivering vitamin C to the skin is naturally, with foods and oils that are high in the vitamin. Blackberry seed oil, rose hip seed oil, sea buckthorn oil, passion flower seed oil, pumpkin seed oil, and mango butter will deliver vitamin C to the skin in a stable form that the body can readily use.

Vitamin D, while not found in plants or their oils, does have a synergistic role to play in the skin with the plant oils. Synthesized by cholesterol in the middle layer of the skin through the action of sunlight, application of natural oils enhance absorption of the vitamin in the body. Resist washing immediately after spending time outdoors to increase production and absorption of the vitamin.

Sunscreens, clothing, cloud cover, smog, and far northern latitudes all interfere with production of vitamin D. This production happens year-round only below the 35th parallel; in the US, this includes California south of San Luis Obispo, as well as parts of Arizona, New Mexico, and other southern states. Above that regional line, the vitamin is produced seasonally in the summer months when the sun's rays are long enough for the synthesis to happen.

Vitamin D is a vital nutrient for the health of the body, optimizing calcium absorption in the intestines to maintain bone strength throughout life. In addition, it operates as an anti-inflammatory, regulates the immune system, maintains a strong heart and circulatory system, helps reduce the risk of cancer and diabetes, improves hair growth, aids in recovery from infectious diseases, colds, and flu, improves cognitive function, and helps maintain healthy body weight. The vitamin is a very important contributor to our overall health.

A few foods contain small amounts of the vitamin—some mushrooms, butter, egg yolks, and meats—but only if the animals have had access to sunlight. Fish oils and some fish provide the oil in sufficient quantities to maintain optimum health, and supplements are an alternate form of obtaining the vitamin. But the best source of vitamin D is sunlight on clean skin, without sunscreen, helped by a little natural oil. Using tropical oils topically will aid production and absorption of the vitamin, while protecting the skin from oxidative damage caused by burning sun rays.

Vitamin F is an outdated term for the two essential fatty acids that have been covered previously: alpha-Linolenic acid and linoleic acid.

Vitamin P is an older term for the flavonoids (see previous section).

We have now explained the Wikipedia definition of an oil introduced at the beginning of this book. Truly understanding a subject involves many levels of engagement: mental, functional, experiential, and even emotional. Once contact has occurred, every experience leads to another aspect of greater clarity or deeper understanding. I've said that this book began as a study paper, and while it expanded greatly in scope, length, and presentation, it is still an ongoing project.

The following section is a list of ninety plus oils and their descriptions, botanical names, properties, historical uses, and effects on the skin and body. The section on working with the oils is an introduction to the experiential aspects of their use. The balance of the book is composed of charts, lists, and data on fatty acids and lipids, designed to aid the understanding of the foregoing text. However, the list of oils will never be complete, since more oils are made available each year, and the list has more than doubled in the ten years since this project was initiated.

My recommendation to you is to experience the oils. Use new ones in your cooking, try them on your skin, scent them, whip them, emulsify them and just have a good time with these gifts from mother nature.

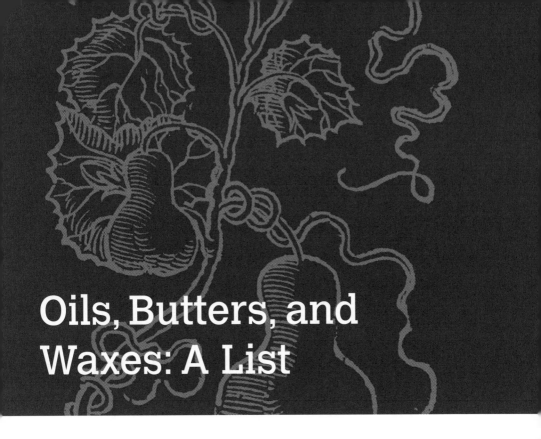

Oils, Butters, and Waxes: A List

Although it features common and not-so-common oils, vegetable butters, and waxes, this list is only a beginning. The market regularly offers up new oils from new sources around the globe, and changing interests in health and natural living also influence the oils that will be popular at any given time. The list of oils available for use is always changing.

Our subject includes the familiar oils: common and excellent standbys such as almond, sunflower, olive, and apricot kernel have been used for years, and are now a standard part of skin and body care. But global travel and immigration have given us new neighbors, with other traditions of skin care and cooking oils, such as argan, tamanu, baobab, neem, acai, and buriti oils. The list is long and growing, and the vocabulary of oils is expanding quickly.

The latest trend in recovering oil is pressing the seeds of common plants to produce new and unusual oils. What was once so much pomace (leftovers after juice or pulp is removed for food) and spread on fields is now being re-invented as a source of new lipids. As an example, tomatoes used for juice, sauce, and commercial foods create large volumes of leftover seed and skin. Though once discarded as pomace, it still contains valuable plant nutrients, and when pressed releases the fatty acids contained in the seeds to create a nourishing new oil: tomato seed oil. Cucumber, blueberry, cranberry, blackberry, and raspberry oils are also now available. Many such fruit and vegetable plants are being pressed for their oil once the juice or pulp has been removed for food. High-volume food processing and suitable equipment makes collection, separation, and pressing of these oils now possible.

Seeds are little engines producing the next generation of plant. For plants to grow, they need nourishment until they can produce their own nutrients by photosynthesis. With water and warmth, a seed will germinate, but it also needs energy. Packed into each seed is concentrated sun energy, ready to be used until the time comes when the seedling can reach for its own sunlight. To grow past the seedling stage, the plant relies on stored light in the form of oil. Imagine the potential number of oils out there; it boggles the mind.

Earlier editions of this book identified 35 oils and their qualities. Since then, completely new oils that did not exist commercially or were not readily available have come on to the market. This edition describes over 90 oils and butters currently available, plus a small section on vegetable waxes and two animal waxes commonly used in skin care.

Organized alphabetically by common name, each listing also includes the Latin botanical binomial. Using the binomial name, a universal identification, avoids the confusion possible with common names. The INCI name for each oil is also included. "INCI" refers to the International Nomenclature of Cosmetic Ingredients, an international standard for all cosmetic ingredients worldwide. In the case of botanical ingredients, the INCI is based on the Latin binomial.

Soaps have their own INCI names, which depend on the oil used. After identifying the type of hydroxide, sodium, or potassium involved, the oil's name is then modified with -ate. *Sodium macadamiate* and *potassium cocoa butterate* for macadamia nut soap or cocoa butter soap, respectively, are two examples.

Our tour of the oils is a global endeavor, beginning with abyssinian oil from the Mediterranean, now grown in Western Canada, and ending with yangu oil from South Africa. The range of oils covers most continents, regions, and climates, from tropical to temperate. Trees, palms, vines, shrubs, berries, annual plants, and perennials make seeds, and many can be pressed for oil.

Abyssinian to Yangu

Abyssinian oil, *Crambe abyssinica,* comes from an oil seed crop native to the Mediterranean, now grown extensively in Western Canada. A member of the cabbage family *Brassica,* abyssinian oil is closely related to rapeseed and mustard. Considered non-edible due to its very high content of erucic acid (22:0), up to 60%, it has been used in manufacturing plastics and lubrication. Oils with high erucic acid content (more than 5%) are restricted from cooking and food products in Canada and the US, as the fatty acid is considered unsuitable for human consumption. Asian cultures don't share the West's reticence, and use oils with erucic acid content (as high as 40%)

freely. In industrial applications, abyssinian oil behaves like mineral oil, but is more biodegradable.

Abyssinian oil is somewhat new to the cosmetics market, with unique properties compared to oils with shorter fatty acid chains. 70 to 75% of abyssinian oil fatty acids are 20 carbons long or longer, making them exceptionally stable and resistant to oxidation. The oil's unusual qualities of lightness, and the ability to penetrate the skin quickly, stem from the high percentage of very-long-chain unsaturated fatty acids. The feel of the oil on the skin is rich and odorless, and the oil absorbs easily. Abyssinian oil replaces lost skin lipids, easing dryness and improving softness and texture. With its long chains of carbon, abyssinian oil is often used in hair care for its non-oily feel and texture.

INCI — *Crambe Abyssinica Seed Oil*

Acai oil, *Euterpe oleracea (a'-se)*, also called the *assai palm*, a native of Brazil and Central and South America, is a member of the botanical family that includes saw palmetto. The South American native population has used the dark purple, grape-sized berries for its nutrients and oil for generations. Nourishing and energizing, the small dark kernels produce oil that is prized for its antioxidant and anti-inflammatory properties. The high content of phytochemicals includes flavanols, vitamins B1, B2, B3, E, and C, with the minerals calcium and potassium as well as proteins. Acai berries have an impressive fatty acid profile, with high percentages of oleic acid (55%) and linoleic acid (45%).

A significant source of anthocyanins (more than in red wine grapes, one of the most recognized sources of these antioxidants), acai oil protects the skin against free radical damage. High in nutrients, emollience, and moisturizing properties, the oil is especially helpful for mature skin, and used in anti-aging

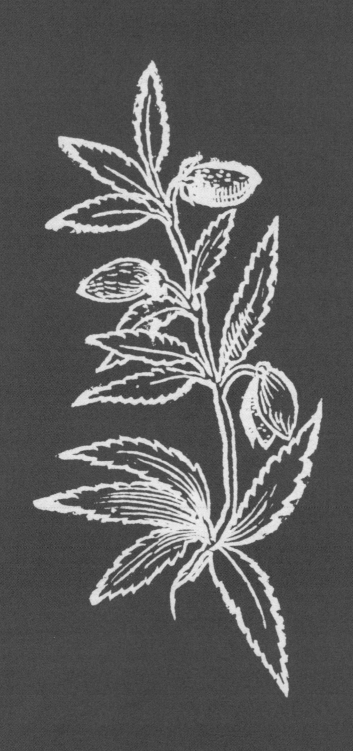

treatments. Nutritionally dense, rich in amino acids, linoleic acid, minerals, and vitamins, the oil helps correct skin conditions like eczema and psoriasis. With a relatively high content of linoleic acid, it also penetrates the skin quickly and deeply. Acai is often used as a carrier oil for aromatherapy and massage, and on swellings. Oils high in plant nutrients, like acai, are shown to help fight cell mutations and unwanted cell proliferation.

INCI—*Euterpe oleracea Fruit Oil*

Almond oil, *Amygdalus communis,* pressed from the common nut, is emollient and mild, a light and nutritious oil for the skin. Quite stable as an unsaturated oil, it is predominantly composed of monounsaturated oleic acid, and also serves as a rich source of linoleic acid, up to between 20 and 30% in some varieties. This oil is also rich in vitamin E (approximately 10 IUs per ounce), squalene, glycosides, and beta-sitosterol—all compounds to soothe the skin and keep it nourished.

Sweet almond oil rates highly in its ability to retain moisture and prevent trans epidermal water loss through the skin. External use of the oil creates a light occlusive protective film for the stratum corneum, the outermost skin layer. With 70% oleic acid, and 20% linoleic acid, almond oil penetrates the skin at a moderate rate. Phytosterols also provide anti-inflammatory protection and support the barrier function of the skin. Lubricating and conserving, almond oil's emollient properties have been shown to be present several days after application to dry or damaged skin.

INCI—*Amygdalus communis (Almond) Oil*

As a soap-making oil, almond contributes lathering properties and is soothing to the skin. The unrefined oil is highest in the native nutrients found in almonds, and is a good oil for soap and salve making.

⚕ **Almond**

Aloe vera oil, *Aloe barbadensis*, is a composite or composed oil

made of a base oil with aloe extracts added. The oil is not pressed from aloe leaf, the healing part of the plant, as the leaves do not carry lipids in any recoverable quantity. Labeled *aloe oil* for marketing purposes, this can be confusing, since the name implies the oil is from aloe. Since this is a composed oil, when used in soap the recipe calculations must be based on the SAP value of the underlying base oil. The INCI name included here is for soybean oil, but aloe extracts can be added to coconut oil, almond oil, or any other readily available oil. The SAP value for calculating soap recipes will vary depending on the base oil used.

INCI—*Glycine soya oil, Aloe barbadensis*

Andiroba oil, *Carapa guianensis*, is in the same family as the

Neem tree, *Meliaceae*. The oils are similar and share active properties. Andiroba, a native of Brazil's Amazon basin, is used by the local population for treating skin conditions. Able to heal cuts and wounds, andiroba oil also treats insect bites, and acts as an insecticidal oil on the skin. Lightly solid at room temperature, it is a light oil, melting easily and readily absorbed into the skin layers. Its 50% monounsaturated oleic acid is balanced by 28% palmitic and 11% linoleic acids.

Andiroba oil contains anti-inflammatory properties, helping to increase circulation in the skin. High in limonoids and triterpenes, andiroba oil is helpful for easing inflammation, and treating painful joints, tension, and tightness in the body. Able to reduce swelling and relieve pain, it is also anti-viral, anti-fungal, and anti-bacterial. Along with oleic, palmitic, and linoleic acids, it is also made up of small amounts of palmitoleic and alpha-Linolenic acids. Andiroba is moisturizing and skin rejuvenating, able to treat skin conditions like acne, eczema, and psoriasis. A useful well-rounded oil.

INCI — *Carapa guianensis (Andiroba) Seed oil*

Apricot kernel oil, *Prunus armeniaca*, is an oil very similar to

almond with a lighter, softer touch. Its linoleic acid content is higher than almond, making up 34% of the oil. Apricot kernel oil is excellent for mature skin due to its emollient, nourishing, and revitalizing properties. A generous vitamin E content provides free radical protection from oxidation of cell membranes, while the phytosterol beta-sitosterol is anti-inflammatory, soothing irritation and supporting the protective barrier function of the skin. Unrefined apricot oil is very light and can have a nutty marzipan/almond scent. In soap, it has properties similar to almond oil, providing good lather and excellent skin-nourishing properties.

The kernels of apricots have an unusual property, possessing the highest concentration of nitrilosides in the plant world. Nitrilosides, also called vitamin B-17 or laetrile, have been promoted as a cancer preventative plant compound, and are a part of laetrile therapy for treatments of cancer-related conditions. Although this treatment has not been proven scientifically, many claim its benefits. The use of apricot kernel oil in cancer salves, in skin treatments for those with high risk for cancer and for cancer patients, *could* be beneficial. An interesting book for exploring this subject is Ingrid Naiman's *Cancer Salves.*

INCI — *Prunus armeniaca (Apricot) Kernel Oil*

INCI Soap — *Sodium Apricot Kernelate*

Argan oil, *Argania spinosa,* is pressed from the nuts of the indigenous argan tree, a native of Morocco, where it is a traditional food and oil. Historically the fruit was eaten by the local livestock, with the goats actually climbing into the trees to munch on the nuts. Google "argan goats in trees" for some amazing images. In this traditional method of collection, the kernels first passed through the goats after they had eaten the argan fruit, and were then collected from the ground and pressed for oil. As the oil has grown in popularity, more modern methods of collection and processing the nuts are in use. Indigenous to Morocco, argan trees are adapted to harsh dry desert conditions and perform similar protective functions for the skin, sealing moisture in while protecting against harsh sun, air, and high temperatures.

Light and capable of penetrating the skin without feeling greasy, argan is an excellent oil for use in skin care and for treating problem skin. Predominately monounsaturated oleic acid and polyunsaturated linoleic acid, it is emollient and nourishing. Generously supplied with vitamin E, polyphenols, squalene, and carotenes, the antioxidant compounds protect the skin against free radical damage. Considered anti-aging, anti-inflammatory, and moisturizing, argan oil can be used directly as a massage oil or added to skin care combinations. Lovingly referred to as *Liquid Gold* by the people of Morocco for its health-giving properties, its reputation is now expanding around the globe.

INCI— *Argania Spinosa (Argan) Nut Oil*

INCI Soap— *Sodium Argannate*

Avocado oil, *Persea gratissima,* is highly nutritious and therapeutic for skin care. It comes from what's known as a "fruiting body," the flesh that surrounds the seed, similar to olives. Pressed from the soft fleshy fruit and used for cooking and eating, skin care, and cosmetics, avocado is a popular oil. Less common is oil pressed from the hard pit, which is used exclusively for skin care due to its reportedly bitter taste. With 20% essential unsaturated linoleic acid and a generous 12% of rare palmitoleic acid, it nourishes skin and supports the health of the stratum corneum.

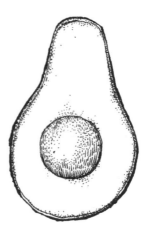

Avocado oil has an impressive percentage of unsaponifiable compounds. These include vitamins A, B, and E, proteins, and amino acids, as well as a small amount of the phospholipid lecithin. The oil's action increases water-soluble collagen content in the middle layer of skin, the dermis. When lacking soluble collagen, the skin appears aged and thin. The phytosterol content of avocado oil supports the collagen and skin structures, helping prevent age spots and cell wall weakening, while calming inflammation, regenerating tissues, and protecting the barrier functions of the skin.

Avocado is one of several oils high in carotenoids that provide natural protection against the effects of ultraviolet rays of the sun. Protecting and regenerating, the oil is easily absorbed. For those with sensitive or damaged skin, it will help to repair and soften skin tissues, healing scaly skin and scalp.

INCI— *Persea gratissima (Avocado) Oil*

The unrefined oil has an especially high unsaponifiable fraction, up to 11%, and is very thick and green. The color will tint soap or cream a strong shade of green or gray, depending on the proportion used. However, avocado oil works well in soap, speeding saponification and making a hard and therapeutic bar.

INCI Soap — *Sodium Avocadate*

Babassu oil, *Orbignya oleifera* or *Attalea speciosa,* comes from a

tree that has two botanical names as of this writing. Pale yellow to white, the tropical solid oil/butter is from the babassu palm that grows in the Amazon region of South America. Cusi, the oil's indigenous name, is used for cooking, as medicine, for skin care, and in beverages. In Brazil, the fallen nuts are collected from August to November and broken open with axes by the "babassu breakers," mostly women, who process the nuts into oil.

Babassu is one of a few oils containing significant percentages of the medium-chain saturated fatty acids, including lauric acid. The oil absorbs well, melting on contact with the skin, a characteristic of medium-length fatty acid carbon chains. Its lauric, caprylic, and capric acids provide the skin-conditioning, anti-microbial, and anti-viral properties of the medium-chain saturated fatty acids. Babassu can be used in ways similar to coconut oil, having a similar feel and fatty acid composition and lacking only the lovely coconut scent.

In addition to its lauric acid content, babassu has 15% myristic acid (14:0). Myristic acid is a beneficial saturated fatty acid with anti-inflammatory properties, and is made by the skin's sebum. It's just two carbon atoms longer than lauric acid (16:0), and more closely matches the actions of lauric acid than the long chain fatty acid stearic. The oil, while saturated, melts easily, quickly penetrating tissues, overcoming dryness, and protecting the outermost skin layer. High in vitamin E and phytosterols, its antioxidant and anti-inflammatory properties are protective and nourishing.

INCI— *Orbignya Oleifera (Babassu) Oil*

The lauric acid content of babassu oil produces excellent lather in soap, as does coconut, with its similar fatty acid profile.

INCI Soap— *Sodium Babassate*

Baobab oil, *Adansonia digitata,* is known across the African continent and has its own botanical family, *Bombacaceae.* Its name in Swahili is *Mbuyu.* Sometimes also called the "upside down tree" because of its unusual shape, the trees can live for 6,000 years. The baobab is indigenous to eastern and southern Africa, and has been used by the native population for centuries. Its interesting fatty acid profile includes a balance of oleic and linoleic acids, around 32% each, with stabilizing palmitic acid around 25% and 3% alpha-Linoleic acid. A stable oil, it has a shelf life of two-plus years when stored well, and will help produce products resistant to oxidation and rancidity.

Even refined baobab oils contain an array of vitamins and phytonutrients, including vitamins A, D, and E. The oil has significant regenerating, moisturizing, and toning properties, and is able to restructure and soften the skin. Baobab oil aids mature skin care by improving elasticity of the tissues and supporting collagen health. Able to soothe cuts, burns, and alleviate painful skin conditions, it is excellent for use in healing ointments made for damaged skin. It is also used for before and after sun care, and repair of acne and rosacea conditions.

INCI— *Adansonia digitata (Baobab) Seed Oil*

Ben oil, or Behen oil, see **Moringa**

Blackberry seed oil, *Rubus fruticosus,* is a member of the prolific rose family. It has a feel similar to other members of the family, with a lightness that is easily and deeply absorbed. It is high in a number of phyto-nutrients and essential fatty acids. Rich in linoleic acid (60%) and alpha-Linolenic acid (15%), the oil will deeply nourish the skin with necessary essential fatty acids. Vitamin E tocopherol and tocotrienol compounds, beta-sitosterol and carotenoid, and lutien are also anti-inflammatory and free radical-scavenging, soothing, and protecting to all layers while nourishing the skin.

But blackberry seed oil really stands out for its generous vitamin C content. Vitamin C is known to help slow skin aging when present in skin tissues, and supports the production of collagen. Blotchy areas, wrinkling, and large pores are improved or prevented with this vitamin. The vitamin C content in blackberry seed oil is a stable source for use in products or directly on the skin. The synthetic water-soluble vitamin is notoriously unstable, especially when combined with water-based materials and held over time, but the natural forms here deliver the benefits directly to the skin. The problems of irritation found with synthetic forms of vitamin C are also avoided when natural sources are used. Massaged into the face, blackberry seed oil is soft-feeling, gentle, and soaks in quickly. This unsaturated oil has a two-year shelf life when stored well, thanks to its generous phytonutrient content.

INCI — *Rubus Fruticosus (Blackberry) Seed Oil*

Black cumin, see Nigella

Black currant seed oil, *Ribes nigrum,* is from the fruit of the *Ribes* genus, native to England and northern Europe. The fruit and the oil are an important source of vitamin C. Black currant seed is also one of the

few oils high in gamma-Linolenic acid (GLA), containing up to 20%. This is an important unsaturated fatty acid for the skin and body. Vital to healthy functioning of cells, GLA is a building block molecule of the immune system. As a fundamental nutrient, the body does not need to modify GLA before using it. Skin absorption is a means to providing the nutrient to the body in addition to diet.

The ability to improve elasticity, calm inflammation, and care for sensitive skin and conditions of eczema and psoriasis makes black currant seed an important oil for skin care. It is capable of penetrating the tissues easily, supplying fatty acids and nutrients to joints and muscles, and helping to repair the results of stress on the body. The GLA, vitamin C, and phytosterols in black currant seed oil support collagen and skin regeneration and act as anti-aging agents to moisturize and maintain skin tone. The oil is also excellent for treating dry and devitalized skin.

INCI — *Ribes nigrum (Black Currant) Seed Oil*

Black seed, see Nigella

Blueberry seed oil, *Vaccinium corymbosum, or V. myrtillus.*
Known for its extremely high levels of antioxidants, blueberry seed oil measures up to the nutritional reputation of the fruit. A newer product, the oil is light and pale-green with a delicate blueberry scent. Very high in both essential fatty acids, linoleic (40%) and alpha-Linolenic (25%), it can deeply nourish skin layers. Rich in phytosterols, carotenoids, and vitamin E, the oil is potent even when used in low percentages. Blueberry oil is able to effectively deliver nutritional and active benefits to protect the stratum corneum and repair damage, including scar tissue. It can also regenerate tissues, smooth fine lines, and increase elasticity of the skin.

Of particular interest is its high content of vitamin E compounds, tocopherols and tocotrienols. These balanced natural antioxidant constructs are readily used by the skin for combating free radical damage. The very unsaturated tocotrienols are mobile and active, more so than the tocopherols. Able to move rapidly to block or neutralize damage from free radical activity, they are particularly beneficial for skin health and repair, slowing down aging processes and protecting health.

INCI— *Vaccinium Corymbosum (Blueberry) Seed Oil*

Borage seed oil, *Borago officinalis*, is pressed from the seeds of

the beautiful, delicate borage flower. The oil has the highest content of gamma-Linolenic acid, GLA (25%), of any oil, including evening primrose and black currant seed. The high GLA content helps regenerate, firm, and rejuvenate the skin's barrier function, decreasing water loss and maintaining the skin's elasticity. Along with beneficial GLA, borage seed oil contains linoleic acid (35%), helping to prevent wrinkles and premature aging, and fighting loss of skin elasticity and dryness.

A broad range of phytochemicals and nutrients stimulate cellular activity in the skin while providing anti-inflammatory actions effective against pain in the joints and soft tissues. Ferulic acid, an antioxidant more effective than vitamin E, protects and soothes damage caused by sun and weather. This is an astringent oil, and the tannins create a dry feeling on the skin, while also calming redness and minimizing pore size. Ellagic acid supports the production of collagen, preventing its breakdown and regenerating skin cells.

INCI— *Borago Officinalis (Borage) Seed Oil*

INCI Soap— *Sodium Boragate*

Black Currant ›

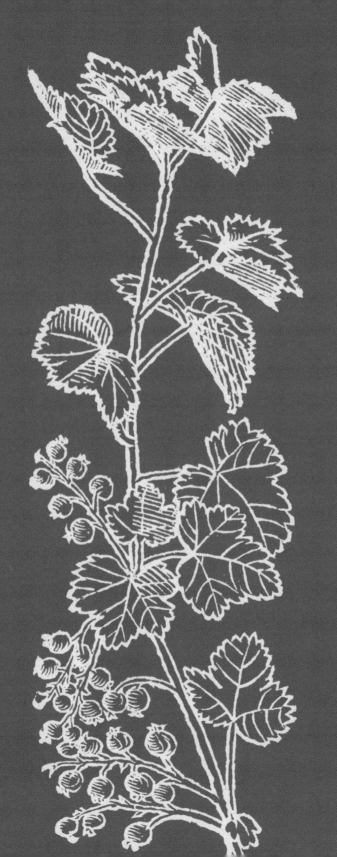

Brazil nut oil, *Bertholletia excelsa,* is an extremely large tree of the Amazonian basin. The nuts and oil are used in cooking and skin and hair care. Indigenous to the Amazon, there is only one species of insect, a bee, that pollinates the fruit. These very large trees produce equally large grapefruit-sized nut casings of four-plus pounds each. They are said to come crashing down to the ground from branches high in the trees. The brazil nuts are arranged inside the casings like segments of an orange. Native people burn the nuts for light, similar to the way Hawaiian kukui are used.

Brazil nut is another oil with an unusual fatty acid profile and is similar to baobab. With nearly equal proportions of oleic and linoleic acids and with palmitic acid providing a stable and protective lesser percentage, it is semi-solid and thick, an oil that liquefies easily. Brazil nuts and oil contain selenium, an antioxidant trace mineral that along with vitamins A and C plays a role in maintaining the skin's stratum corneum. The selenium content helps maintain skin elasticity, protecting against UV rays and repairing damage from sun and environmental stresses. Moisturizing, banishing dryness, and supporting and protecting the tissues of the skin, brazil nut oil is a valuable ingredient for skin care.

INCI — *Bertholletia excelsa (Brazil) Nut Oil*

Broccoli seed oil, *Brassica oleracea italica,* is roughly 50% omega-9 erucic acid (C22:1), a very-long-chain unsaturated fatty acid. A member of the cabbage, or *Brassica* family, broccoli seed oil moisturizes with stable, non-greasy, yet effective action. The very-long-chain fatty acids help protect against damage from excess sun. And broccoli seed oil makes an excellent hair conditioning treatment, smoothing dry frizzy hair without leaving an oily feel.

Sulforaphane, a compound associated with the cabbage family, provides

UV protection by stimulation of protective enzymes. Broccoli seeds are especially high in sulforaphane and able to stimulate the production of the enzyme glutathione, a co-enzyme antioxidant that all cells make. Glutathione acts by continuously protecting cells, neutralizing and eliminating toxins and free radicals. Glutathione also stimulates anti-inflammatory actions in capillaries, reducing the effects of rosacea by slowing, even halting, new growth in the fine blood vessels of the face.

Oils with very-long-chain unsaturated fatty acids, 20 carbons atoms or more, have a silicone-like feeling, thick and viscous yet protective. Silicone is used in body care to add sheen and luster to products. Broccoli seed oil is a natural alternative to synthetic silicone, providing the desired qualities and penetrating the cells without leaving an oily residue behind. The oil is useful for hair care and non-oily skin care. Unless highly refined, it has a mild scent of sulfur, like cooked cabbage, and is pale green. When used in low dilutions, the scent can be overcome by other ingredients.

INCI — *Brassica oleracea italica (Broccoli) Seed Oil*

Buriti oil, *Mauritia flexuosa*, is known as the moriche palm from

Brazil and the Amazon basin (*Buriti* in Brazil means "tree of life"). Very deep red-orange, the oil is the richest source of carotenoids and beta-carotene, being more generously endowed than even carrots. Red-orange carotenoids and polyphenolic compounds have the ability to provide a great deal of protection against damaging UV sun rays. By preventing and repairing damage from excess sun exposure, the pro-vitamin A carotenes and other antioxidants provide important protective actions by neutralizing and halting the free radical damage that too much sun can cause. Rich in vitamin E tocopherols, buriti oil restores moisture in the skin cells, preventing oxidative damage and skin degeneration.

Buriti oil's natural gifts help heal wounds and prevent excessive scarring in skin tissues. The unsaturated fatty acids, primarily oleic acid, help to rejuvenate, moisturize, and rebuild the skin, maintaining its elasticity. The deep color can stain cloth and porous surfaces, but does not stain skin, soaking in or washing off easily. Used in small amounts in cosmetics and high-end skin care, buriti oil will color formulas a beautiful yellow that represents the very nourishing and rejuvenating properties in the product.

INCI — *Mauritia flexuosa (Buriti) Seed Oil*

Camelina oil, *Camelina sativa*, a native of Europe and Central Asia, is grown as an oil seed crop. With a variety of names—*wild flax, linseed dodder, German sesame*, and *Siberian oilseed*—we get a feel for the crop's wide range and tradition as an important food source. Archeological evidence shows the crop has been in cultivation for over 3,000 years. A member of the *Brassica* family, camelina oil was used in lamps for light and is eaten as food for its high content of alpha-Linolenic acid (40%). With the oil's high nutritional content, it has also been used as a substitute for flax oil. As a member of the cabbage family, its relatively low erucic acid content is only 2%, naturally. Only in recent decades has camelina come to the New World, and become an agricultural crop on the North American continent. In Europe, it is sold under the name "Gold of Pleasure."

With camelina's high omega-3 fatty acid (40%), omega-6 (22%), and monounsaturated fatty acids (30%), it is a surprisingly stable oil. Considerable amounts of vitamin E tocopherols and other anti-oxidants protect the oil against oxidation. With an omega-3 to omega-6 ratio of 2 to 1, the oil is able to help balance dietary imbalances of EFAs. Oils high in both essential fatty acids are quickly and easily absorbed into the skin. Camelina is especially beneficial for topical use, and is a nutritious oil for use in the kitchen. It has a two-year shelf life, which is very unusual for one so high in omega-3 fatty acids.

INCI— *Camelina sativa Seed Oil*

Camellia oil or tea seed oil, *Camellia sasanqua, C. seninsis, C. oleifera,* is pressed from the seeds of the winter-blooming shrub of the camellia or tea family. The different varieties produce similar but distinct oils for cooking and skin care. Camellia oil, known as *tsubaki oil,* has been popular in Japan for cooking, skin, and hair care for thousands of years. It is said to be responsible for the peachy skin and long, curved nails of Japanese women.

Camellia oil is high in monounsaturated oleic acid (80%), giving it excellent skin- and hair-conditioning properties. The oil does not clog pores or leave an oily feel, due to tannins present in the seeds. An astringent oil, it is a good choice compared to other high-oleic oils for oily or problem skin. As a dry cooling oil, it also helps with prevention and repair of scarring. Able to rejuvenate and maintain moisture in the skin, its protective polyphenols, vitamins A, B, C, and E, and other antioxidants also protect the skin from UV and environmental exposure, arresting the effects of free radical damage. As camellia oil is easily absorbed, its plant-derived squalene nourishes and supports the skin. Traditionally used in Japan, camellia oil is becoming increasingly popular in the West.

INCI— *Camellia sasanqua Seed Oil*

Canola oil, *Brassica napus/campestris.* The name "canola" is an acronym for "Canada Oil Low Acid" (Can O L A). Originally called rapeseed, or LEAR (Low-Erucic Acid Rapeseed), the name canola was designed to make the oil more appealing on the market. Another high oil-producing plant of the

Brassica family, "low acid" refers to the reduced erucic acid that has been bred out of (or bred to very low levels) in the seeds. It was once thought that erucic acid was damaging to the heart muscle and so unsuitable for human consumption. Canola oil remains controversial, and conflicting reports on its health benefits will no doubt continue.

Canola is high in oleic acid and contains the essential fatty acids linoleic and alpha-Linolenic acids. Being intensively farmed, much of the crop is heavily sprayed and genetically modified. Canola is usually highly refined, which damages nutritional properties. Organic canola oil can be found on the market and is produced primarily for food products.

INCI — *Brassica campestris*

Canola oil's low price makes it useful for soap-making. Finding an organic version avoids agricultural contaminants and GMOs (genetically modified organisms). As a soap-making oil, canola is one of the lowest in saturated fatty acids, which will make it slow to saponify. In smaller quantities and combined with a balance of saturated oils, it will provide proteins and moisturizing properties in the soap mixture.

INCI Soap — *Sodium Canolate*

Carrot seed oil, *Daucus carota*, is cold-pressed from the seed as

a fixed oil and should not be confused with the essential oil distilled from the seeds. The same seed source can create two very different products. Carrot seeds have sufficient fatty acids for pressing as a fixed oil and enough volatile aromatic compounds to make an essential oil. Both products are beneficial for use on the skin to nourish and repair skin tissues.

Carrot seed fixed oil is dark green with a green scent and extremely bitter taste. Exceptionally rich in beta carotene provitamin A, it also provides UV protection. In addition, its vitamin E and natural mineral content make the oil highly nutrient-dense. Healing for dry, chapped, and cracked skin, carrot seed oil helps to balance moisture in the tissues. High in the phytosterols, stigmasterol, beta-sitosterol, and beta carotene, the oil is protective and healing. It is also used as a conditioner for hair.

INCI — *Daucus carota (Carrot) Seed Oil*

Carrot root oil or helio carrot, *Daucus carota*, includes cold-pressed compounds found in the root of the carrot, which are macerated with a carrier oil to extend and carry them. It is also extracted as a CO2 *total*, which includes the whole of the plant compounds including waxes, nutrients, and essential oils. This is then extended with a fixed oil, as carrot root oil does not have its own fatty acid profile, instead adopting that of its carrier oil. Similar to aloe oil, the beneficial compounds are carried in the base oil. Jojoba, soy, and canola are the base oils often used.

Helio carrot, a commercial name for the root oil, is rich in mixed carotenoids and provitamin A compounds, as indicated by its deep yellow-orange color. There are over 600 identified carotenoids, antioxidants that are easily assimilated by the body, found in carrots. The root oil includes many of these, including beta-carotene, lycopene, alpha carotene, lutein, canthaxanthin, and zeaxanthin—all powerful antioxidants.

Carrot root oil protects against sunburns by absorbing UV rays while nourishing skin cells and preventing damage associated with sun exposure. Through their antioxidant activity, carotenoids in the oil are photo-protective of cells and tissues. These antioxidant properties protect both the structure and function of the cell membranes that are shielded against ultraviolet rays and environmental pollutants, preventing degeneration and premature aging. Carotenoids have also been shown to inhibit the proliferation of certain types of cancer cells.

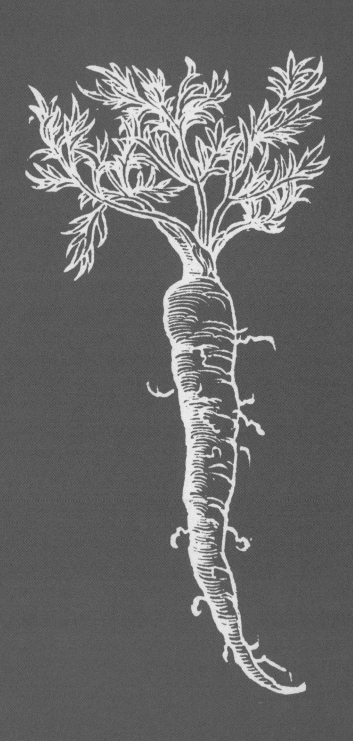

INCI— *(base oil) and Daucus carota (Carrot) Root Oil*

Alternate INCI— *Glycine Soja (Soybean) Oil (and) Daucus carota sativa (Carrot) Root Extract (and) Tocopherol*

Castor oil, Ricinus communis, is also called *Palma Christi*, or "hand of Christ," a reference to its healing abilities, which have been used for over 4,000 years. Edgar Cayce recommended castor oil often in his trance healing, successfully treating many people. The ancient Egyptian Ebers Papyrus also contains information about the uses and benefits of castor oil. Ancient and modern Greece, India, Persia, China, and Africa use castor oil for treating the body via skin applications. Along with olive oil, castor oil has been used for millennia and figures prominently in many healing traditions. The oil is not for internal consumption, as it causes unpleasant gastric upset and is used as a laxative.

Castor oil differs from other eighteen-carbon fatty acid-dominant oils by being thick and viscous yet easily absorbed by the skin. The unique ricinoleic acid is high in the oil, at 90%, and has an unusual fatty acid structure. Ricinoleic acid has a hydroxyl group (-OH) on the twelfth carbon, or sixth carbon from the methyl, free, end of the chain. This structure causes ricinoleic acid to be more polar, water-accepting, than other fatty acids.

The increased ability of castor oil to penetrate the skin allows it to carry nutrients into the body by external application. Castor oil is taken up by the skin, where its properties stimulate and diffuse into the body and organs. Likewise, castor oil can deliver unwanted chemicals into the body, so care needs to be exercised when using it with ingredients that may not be natural.

Castor oil packs placed on the liver and abdominal area are a common method of alternative treatment for a number of conditions, including constipation, liver congestion, and inflamation. They are also used to increase immune function. Placed thickly on the skin, the oil is covered with a cloth,

⟨ **Carrot**

kept warm, and left for thirty to forty minutes a day. Treatment may last a few days, or extend over a period of weeks or months for chronic conditions. The blood and lymph are activated and movement of the fluids within the body releases toxic elements stored in the liver and other tissues. By stimulating the immune system, the body normalizes and ideally returns to a healthy state. Castor oil also helps to minimize scarring when used in treatments for cuts, wounds, and other traumas to the skin. It is soothing and lubricating, acting as a humectant and drawing moisture to it to hydrate the skin.

INCI — *Ricinus communis (Castor) Seed Oil*

When it comes to making soap, the molecular makeup of ricinoleic acid is unusual due to the uncommon placement of the hydroxyl group on the fatty acid chain. More hydroxide ions are needed to make soap than its SAP (saponification) value indicates. Too high a percentage of castor oil in a recipe will produce a soft transparent soap, but used at less than 15% in a recipe, it adds a lovely soft lather to bar soaps. When saponified with potassium hydroxide (KOH), castor oil makes an excellent but non- to low-lathering shampoo for the hair.

INCI Soap — *Sodium Castorate or Sodium Ricinoleate*

Caulophyllum Inophyllum, *Caulophyllum inophyllum,* commercially called tamanu and foraha, is an oil pressed from the nuts of a large tropical evergreen tree found throughout the Pacific Basin. The number of common names for the tree reflect its presence throughout the region: beach calophyllum, alexandrian laurel, balltree, beautyleaf, borneo-mahogany, oil tree, indian-laurel, and Indian doomba are a few. Native names for the tree also reflect its universality: it's known as *Tamanu* in Tahiti; *Kamanu or Kamani* in Hawaii; *fetau* in Samoa; and *faraha* in Madagascar. Dilo oil is a

name used in the Pacific region, while tamanu and foraha are names used in commerce. Considered sacred in Tahiti, the tree and all its parts have been used in healing traditions since ancient times.

Books on aromatherapy often include tamanu oil, as it has considerable beneficial effects on the skin. Chemically, it is a fixed oil, not a volatile or essential oil. The oil is referred to as "green gold" and is very thick and dark green, with a pungent but "healing" scent. It is a member of the botanical family *Clusiaceae*, whose other members include mangosteen and St. John's wort.

Tamanu has the usual triglycerides and plant compounds found in many oils, but also has unusual and exceptional properties. In addition to commonly occurring oleic, linoleic, palmitic, and stearic acids, tamanu also contains the wholly new calophyllic fatty acid, as well as glycolipids (lipids with starches attached) and phospholipids. A new phyto compound, calophyllolide, unique to the tree and oil, is strongly anti-inflammatory and a healing agent. With its unusual composition, tamanu oil absorbs deeply into all three layers of the skin, where it has been demonstrated to rapidly regenerate new skin, repair nerves, and diminish scarring. Useful in the treatment of sciatica, rheumatism, and shingles, it is also used to treat eczema, psoriasis, chapping, burns, cracked skin, fissures, and infections. Historically, it is reputed to even treat leprosy. Open wounds and serious breaches of the body have reportedly been repaired with treatment with the oil. It is anti-inflammatory, anti-bacterial, and analgesic, while being non-toxic and non-irritating.

Tamanu is a very thick oil, semi-saturated at room temperature, as are many tropical oils. Rubbed on damp skin, it has a beautiful smooth, silky, non-oily feel. If too liquid, the healing properties have been damaged or refined out. With a strong, not unpleasant nutty scent, it is expensive but well worth the cost as an excellent addition to salves and creams. With its highly therapeutic properties, tamanu oil also makes a therapeutic soap that produces abundant lather on contact with sea water.

INCI — *Caulophyllum inophyllum*

Cherry kernel oil, *Prunus avium*, is pressed from cherry pits.

Cherry kernel oil belongs to the rose family of oils. The oil contains an unusual fatty acid, eleostearic acid (12%), not usually found in oils from the rose family. This fatty acid is found in large quantities in bitter melon seed oil (60%), and tung oil (82%). As a conjugated fatty acid, eleostearic acid plays a role in prostaglandin production in the body, and along with the essential fatty acids, also plays an important part in health regulation. Cherry kernel oil has also been shown to slow tumor growth in animal tests.

Cherry kernel oil is heavier on the skin than other rose family oils because of the properties of the conjugated eleostearic fatty acid. For skin and hair care, the fatty acid creates a protective barrier that minimizes absorption of UV rays. A stable oil, it is richly endowed with the vitamin A and vitamin E compounds alpha, delta, and gamma tocopherols and tocotrienols. The very active and antioxidant tocotrienols are some of the highest of any oil. A balance of the omega-6 and 9 fatty acids gives cherry kernel oil important skin moisturizing and protective properties. Phytosterols and phospholipids also soften and nourish skin cells. Cherry kernel oil, along with other oils from the rose family, is beneficial for the health of the skin and has a place in cosmetics and therapeutic remedies.

INCI — *Prunus Avium (Cherry kernel) Oil*

Chia seed oil, *Salvia hispanica*, is a member of the mint family,

Laminaceae, and native to central Mexico. Chia seeds and oil have been used for centuries for their nutritive and health-sustaining properties by the indigenous people of Mexico and Central America. Tradition has it the Aztecs relied on chia's nourishment for physical strength and mental agility when they went to war.

Chia seeds are exceptionally high in the omega-3 essential fatty acids, up to 60%. Balanced with omega-6 fatty acids (21%), amino acids, vitamins, and minerals including zinc, the seeds and oil are exceptionally nourishing. Natural antioxidant compounds make chia seed oil stable against oxidation, in contrast to flax oil, which readily reacts. The high content of essential fatty acids and stability make chia seed oil a natural for topical use. Anti-inflammatory and antioxidant, chia seed oil is used for treating stubborn skin issues and to prevent scarring. Its high zinc content helps regenerate skin tissues, aiding in the treatment of acne and preventing scarring from the lesions.

INCI—*Salvia hispanica (Chia) Seed oil*

Cocoa butter, *Theobroma cacao,* is the solid fat from the chocolate fruit and bean. Separated during the manufacture of cocoa and other chocolate products, cocoa butter has emollient properties that leave a fine lipid barrier on the skin, preventing moisture loss. Traditionally used during pregnancy to prevent and repair stretch marks, cocoa butter is often found in creams and salves for pregnancy and childbirth.

High in the saturated long-chain stearic and palmitic fatty acids, cocoa butter is very hard at room temperature in temperate climates. Not easily absorbed, and classified as an occlusive ingredient, cocoa butter protects the skin with a physical barrier against water loss. Because of its highly saturated occlusive properties, it is often combined with other oils. Melted together with coconut oil, shea butter, and other saturated and unsaturated oils, cocoa butter makes wonderful salves that are protective and emollient.

INCI— *Theobroma cacao (Cocoa) Seed Butter*

Cocoa butter is a gift to soap-making, as it helps make a hard bar of soap that also nourishes and treats the skin gently. However, too high a saturated oil percentage will produce bars that are very hard, brittle, and have a tendency to crack.

INCI Soap—*Sodium Cocoa Butterate*

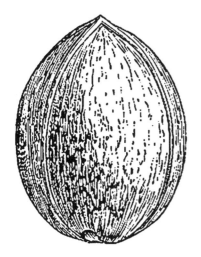 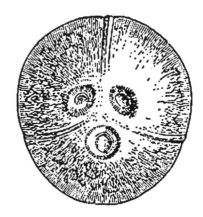

Coconut oil, Cocos nucifera, as a commercial product, has evolved

a great deal over the past decade in its uses and reputation. Unique characteristics make it a valuable oil for food and cooking, health, skin care, cosmetic manufacturing, and soap-making.

Lauric acid, a medium-chain saturated fatty acid, makes up close to 50% of coconut oil. Benefits for the body include lauric acid's conversion to monolaurin, a compound able to destroy viruses and kill harmful bacteria and protozoa. Medium-chain fatty acids are also easier on the digestive process than longer-chained fatty acids and are assimilated more easily by the body. Increasingly popular in the kitchen, coconut oil as a saturated fat withstands high heat when used for cooking.

Coconut oil and cocoa butter combined work well together in preparations for sun-tanning, with their tropical sources and saturated properties. Fifty years ago, before sun exposure became suffused with fear and anxiety, coconut oil and cocoa butter were the oils of choice for the darkest tans. Oils produced from plants grown in the tropics contain compounds that protect the skin from the sun's rays, while allowing natural vitamin D formation to take place in the skin layers. Used in preparations for the prevention of stretch marks, the oil helps the skin grow and expand without tearing. Where palms are indigenous, coconut oil is used for skin and hair care and in cooking. As a saturated oil, it has softening, moisturizing, and film-forming properties to protect the skin.

INCI — Cocos Nucifera (Coconut) Oil

Coconut oil has great value and versatility in making soap, helping to produce excellent bars. Liquefying at 76°F, its commercial name is "Coconut 76." Extracted from copra, the dried meat of coconuts, the oil is inexpensive. Commercial soap manufacturers use about 20% coconut oil in addition to tallow for its lathering and moisturizing properties. The lauric acid content creates abundant lather even when soap is used in cold seawater. The best soaps are formulated with only 50% saturated oils, or the bars can be drying and harsh on the skin. Combined with a variety of unsaturated oils, coconut oil will produce a great soap.

INCI Soap — Sodium Cocoate

Coconut oil, Virgin is oil extracted from the milk and fresh meat of the coconut rather than copra, the dried meat of the nut. Without certifying standards defining the term "virgin" for coconut oil, as there is with olive oil, the quality varies between producers. Quality coconut oils are processed by technology developed in Japan, using a centrifuge and gravity to extract the pure oil without using solvents. Creamy white virgin coconut oil has the aroma of pure coconut and is readily absorbed into the skin, melting on contact. Virgin oils are more expensive than the 76° variety and can be used for soap, but the delicate coconut aroma will not survive exposure to the lye. For production of creams and salves, the virgin oil is valuable.

INCI—*Cocos Nucifera (Coconut) Milk Oil*

Coconut oil, Fractionated begins as the 76°F version mentioned above, but when hydrolyzed under pressure the fatty acids are separated from the glycerol. The capric and caprylic short-chained saturated fatty acids, those liquid at room temperature, are separated and mixed back in with the glycerin, creating a clear liquid oil that never hardens and has an extended shelf life. Fractionated coconut oil is used for making massage oils and creams. Massage therapists are said to like the oil because it has a good "slip" and does not stain towels or clothing.

INCI— *Caprylic/Capric Triglyceride*

Coffee oil, Green, or Roasted, *Coffea arabica,* is pressed from green, raw, or roasted coffee beans grown in tropical regions around the world, including South America, Asia, and Africa, as well as Hawaii. When roasted, coffee beans undergo a transformation that changes the chemical and aromatic properties and gives us the popular beverage many of us can't live without. Both green and roasted beans are pressed for oil and have similar properties and actions on the skin. The roasted oil, if not deodorized, has an herbaceous coffee scent.

The oil from green coffee beans is high in an unusual combination of linoleic and palmitic acid, in equal amounts of about 40%. The balance of polyunsaturated and saturated fatty acids gives the oil the ability to penetrate the tissues quickly while being extremely moisturizing and protective of the skin surface. Smaller amounts of oleic and alpha-Linolenic acid add nourishing elements. Rich in anti-inflammatory phytosterols, including beta-sitosterol, stigmasterol, and campesterol, the oil supports the health of the skin layers and has the ability to regenerate and repair the tissues. Beneficial for conditions of eczema and psoriasis, it moisturizes dry cracked skin and is excellent for mature skin care.

INCI— *Coffea arabica (Coffee) Seed oil*

Corn oil, Maize oil, Zea mays, is pressed from the germ of

the corn seed, the staple grain of the Native Americans. Corn oil is ubiquitous in grocery aisles and the brand Mazola, for maize, is a main producer. Not usually included in lists of skin care oils, it is most often used as an edible oil. As another crop with heavy GMO production, organic forms are available from the grain grown in Europe. The unrefined oil is a vibrant yellow and has the flavor and aroma of corn.

INCI— *Zea Mays (Corn) Oil*

For soap-making, corn oil is relatively inexpensive even for the organic variety. High in linoleic acid (50%) and oleic acid (30%), it is best balanced with saturated oils for a hard long-lasting bar of soap.

INCI Soap— *Sodium cornate*

Cranberry seed oil, Vaccinium macrocarpon, has nearly equal

ratios of omega-3, omega-6, and omega-9 fatty acids, making it an excellent oil for skin conditioning. In addition to its balanced fatty acid profile, cranberry seed oil is deeply yellow, indicating the presence of provitamin A carotenoids containing antioxidant properties that protect the polyunsaturated fatty acids. Cranberry seed oil belongs to the same botanical family as blueberry, and has a similar composition of phytonutrients and antioxidant compounds beneficial for skin and body health.

Richly endowed with nutrients, including polyphenols, carotenes, quercetin, anthocyanidins, and proanthocyanidins, cranberry seed oil is especially protective against oxidation and free radical damage. The impressive combination of plant nutrients provides stability in spite of its ample polyunsaturated and essential fatty acid content. Tannins keep the oil light-feeling on the skin, and provide antibacterial properties. Beta-Sitosterol eases the redness and itching from inflammation and repairs and regenerates tissues.

Vitamin E tocopherols and tocotrienols are active against free radical damage. Phytosterols and phospholipids help the skin remain elastic and flexible, protecting collagen and skin tissues. Vitamin A aids skin health by guarding against free radical damage and supporting elastin and collagen formation, while helping improve skin conditions where blemishes or acne are persistent. Phyto compounds nourish and condition the skin, providing relief from dryness and scaling, and itchy, irritated conditions. As a specialty oil added to serums and therapeutic applications, it is light and absorbs into the skin fairly quickly.

INCI — *Vaccinium macrocarpon (Cranberry) Seed Oil*

Cucumber seed oil, *Cucumis Sativus*, pressed from dried cucumber seeds, has a fresh aroma and pale, clear yellow color. Unusually high in phytosterols, compounds that strengthen the skin's barrier function, the oil helps maintain moisture levels and elasticity in the skin. High in omega-6 linoleic acid (65%), cucumber seed oil is helpful for a wide range of

skin conditions, including eczema and dermatitis. Its ability to supplement skin deficient in linoleic acid helps rebuild a damaged barrier function. The oil nourishes deeply, and promotes regeneration of the cells of the skin.

The vitamin E complex of both tocopherols and tocotrienols enables cucumber seed oil to actively protect against free radical damage and revitalize skin damaged by sun and weather. Vitamin C and antioxidants aid blood flow, reducing puffy, strained areas with regular use. Similar to cucumber slices placed on puffy eyes, the oil can be used around the eye area to reduce swelling. Anti-inflammatory phytosterols calm burns and blemishes and nourish tissues. With its high silica content, cucumber oil is strengthening to skin and especially the hair, providing structure and support. Cucumber seed oil is a stable oil, highly moisturizing, and absorbs into the skin quickly.

INCI — *Cucumis Sativus (Cucumber) Oil*

Daikon radish seed oil, *Raphanus sativus*, is a new oil on

the market and another from the *Brassica* or cabbage family. Similar to broccoli seed oil, daikon radish oil is high in erucic acid (C22:1) at 34%, and gadoleic acid (C20:1) at 10%; both are very-long-chain unsaturated fatty acids. Used as a replacement for silicone functions in personal and hair care products and cosmetics, the very-long-chain fatty acids are well absorbed and fairly stable. With a fatty acid profile similar to the esters of jojoba oil, daikon radish seed oil has similar properties, however a 12% alpha-Linolenic acid content keeps the oil from being as stable as jojoba or other brassica family oils. Daikon radish seed oil has a recommended shelf life of only six months to a year. Tests have shown that the oil improves the barrier function of the skin significantly over a period of hours. Soft-feeling within minutes of application, the skin is moisturized and the oil well-absorbed.

INCI — *Raphanus Sativus (Radish) Seed Oil*

Evening primrose oil, *Oenothers biennis*, known by its
initials EPO, was the first vegetable oil discovered to supply essential fatty
acids, especially gamma linolenic acid (GLA), in sufficient nutritional
quantities to treat disease and overcome deficiencies. Evening primrose oil
contains GLA in the range of 10%. Since this discovery, black currant seed
(15%) and borage seed (25%) oils have been found to supply even greater
quantities of GLA. As the fatty acid responsible for reducing inflammation,
supporting the immune system, and hormonal balance, GLA also helps
maintain healthy skin, nails, and hair. Studies have shown promise in
overcoming eczema and psoriasis with use of the fatty acid. The presence
of the polyphenol gallic acid speeds the healing of burns and wounds,
while catechins are anti-bacterial. The tannins in the oil provide astringent
properties, keeping the oil feeling light on the skin.

Where there is difficulty in converting the essential alpha-Linolenic acid
in the body, oils high in GLA act as a shorthand step, providing the benefits
of this necessary compound directly without need of conversion. On the skin,
EPO provides nourishing and conditioning properties that are taken up by the
tissues, improving the health of the skin layers. The omega-6 polyunsaturated
GLA and linoleic acids, in particular, benefit the skin, as they are easily
absorbed and able to carry their protective and nutritional compounds into
the skin layers.

INCI— *Oenothers biennis (Evening Primrose) Oil*

Flax seed oil, *Linum usitatissimum*, is one of the oldest oil seed
crops grown and has a multitude of uses. Ponder for a moment its Latin
binomial, *usitatissimum*, then its contribution to our evolution and culture:
food, oil, nutritional supplementation, flooring, fiber, paint, ink, and cloth.
Clearly, this is one "useful" plant. The flax plant produces linen from tough

Flax ⧸⟩

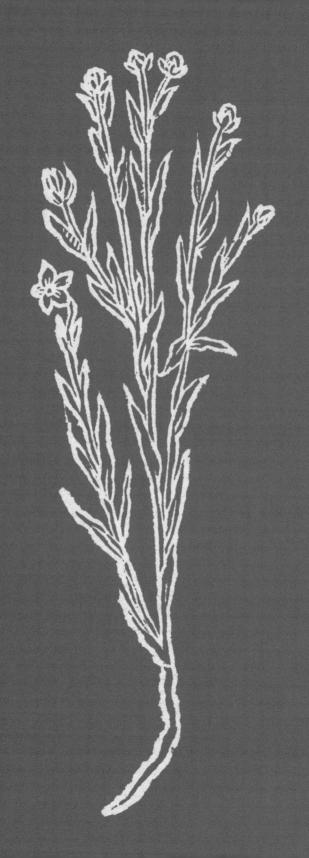

fibers and lipids with widely diverse applications. In industry and non-food uses the oil is known as linseed, from the Latin *Linum*.

Linseed oil, a refined version of flax oil, is highly reactive, readily attracting oxygen to its poly and super-polyunsaturated fatty acids. Used in manufacturing for paints and other industrial applications including flooring, it dries due to its super-unsaturated state when oxygen binds to the unsaturated carbon molecules. The oil becomes sticky and eventually solid. In a food oil, this is called going rancid and means the oil should not be used, while for industrial purposes it is desirable and encouraged.

As a nutritional supplement, unrefined flax seed oil is kept in the refrigerator in dark containers to protect the fatty acids from oxidation. High in the super unsaturated alpha-Linolenic acid with three double bonds, flax is highly reactive to oxygen. This is a plus for its health-giving properties as long as it is protected from becoming rancid before being consumed. The highly unsaturated fatty acids provide the pathway in the body for energy transfers and optimum health. The unrefined food version of flax seed oil is the primary plant source for the omega-3 essential fatty acid alpha-Linolenic acid, and constitutes up to 65% of the oil. Flax seed oil tops all other sources of the fatty acid in the plant world.

INCI— *Linum usitatissimum (Flax) Seed Oil*

Foraha, see Caulophyllum Inophyllum

Gevuina, Chilean Hazelnut, *Gevuina Avellana*, is a beautiful tree from Chile and Argentina and produces small nuts similar to macadamias. Though called Chilean hazelnut, the tree belongs to the same botanical family, *Proteaceae*, as macadamia, and the oils have a similar fatty acid composition. Both oils are high in monounsaturated oleic and palmitoleic

fatty acids, with under 15% polyunsaturates. An important similarity is the content of palmitoleic acid, 20 to 27%, in gevuina oil, which is comparable to macadamia. Gevuina oil is one of the few oils high in this important functional fatty acid found in the skin's sebum. Avocado, macadamia, and sea buckthorn oils are similarly and generously endowed with this valuable fatty acid.

Rich in polyphenol antioxidants, gevuina oil is protective against extreme weather conditions and UV radiation. Vitamin E tocopherols and tocotrienols in the oil quickly penetrate the tissues, protecting all layers against oxidation. Mature skin especially is helped by palmitoleic acid, as the fatty acid represents 20% of the sebum's own production. Protective and repairing, palmitoleic acid supports the skin's own immune system, helping it resist infection and repair wounds. A stable oil, gevuina will last about 18 months with proper care.

INCI — *Gevuina Avellana (Hazelnut) Oil*

Grape-seed oil, *Vitis vinifera*, is pressed from the seeds of grapes

after the juice for food or wine is harvested. Pale green to colorless, the odor and flavor vary depending on the degree of refining. Organic oils tend to be darker and have a light scent, while non-organic oils are often more refined, lighter, or colorless and odorless. Varietal oils from harvesting the Chardonnay, Riesling, Cabernet Sauvignon, and Merlot varieties are available for culinary purposes and can also be used in skin care.

High in vitamin E, the less refined grape-seed oils are pale green and contain natural chlorophyll and antioxidants. Rich in vitamins, minerals, and the flavanol proanthocyanidin, the oil helps strengthen collagen and maintain elastin, the proteins that make up the connective tissue in skin and joints. Grape-seed oil is especially high in the omega-6 essential fatty acid linoleic acid (76%), making it a light oil that penetrates the skin layers. Often used for massage and in body oil combinations for its toning properties, the oil has astringent properties for tightening and toning skin tissues. Grape-seed oil is easily absorbed when used directly on the skin, as a make-up remover, and in skin care products.

Grape-seed oil is often promoted for high heat cooking because of its high smoke point. The oil feels safe to cook with, without all that smoke in the kitchen. The high smoke point is derived from the high polyphenol composition, which keeps the oil from burning, but does not fully protect the linoleic acid from oxidation. There are better oils to use for cooking. Balancing the high linoleic acid omega-6 grape-seed oil with oils high in omega-3 fatty acids makes a healthy addition to the diet.

INCI — *Vitis vinifera (Grape) Seed Oil*

INCI Soap — *Sodium Grapeseedate*

Hazelnut oil, *Corylus aveliana,* is from the hazelnut tree; the nuts

also go by the names filbert or cobnut. Produced in Turkey in large quantities, the tree is also grown in Washington state and Oregon. Primarily used as a food and cooking oil, hazelnut oil is excellent for use on the skin for its astringent properties and generous squalene content.

High in oleic acid (75%), with a smaller amount of linoleic acid (11%), hazelnut oil is able to penetrate the skin with proteins, vitamins including E, minerals, beta-sitosterol, and antioxidants. Hazelnuts' tannin content stimulates skin circulation, while the astringent properties help treat oily or acne-prone skin. Astringency of the tannins treats thread veins, helping to reduce and shrink their size and visibility. As one of the vegetable oils highest in unsaturated fatty acids, it is good for moisturizing and softening. Used in salves and cosmetics, hazelnut oil is readily absorbed and beneficial for skin health.

The hazelnut tree also contains paclitaxel (Taxol), a potent anti-cancer drug first discovered in the Pacific Yew tree. Paclitaxel has been used to treat various cancers, especially of the breast, ovaries, and lung. Studies for its use in psoriasis, multiple sclerosis, Alzheimer's disease, and some kidney diseases are ongoing. Paclitaxel is found in the leaves and stems of the hazelnut tree and in the source of the oil, raw hazelnuts. Its presence helps the tree fight the disease called Eastern Filbert Blight; the higher the tree's content of paclitaxel, the more resistant it is to the blight, studies have found.

INCI— *Corylus aveliana (Hazelnut) Oil*

Hemp seed oil, *Cannabis indica,* and hemp products have become increasingly popular for their many beneficial properties. Hemp and flax, two of the oldest cultivated plants used by mankind, have broad applications and multiple uses. Both are fiber sources for paper and cloth, with linen from flax and canvas and rope from hemp. Their highly nutritious seed oils have also played important roles in our diet and health. Hemp is a sturdy plant, fast-growing and hardy, containing high quality cellulose that makes archival quality paper. Paper made from the fibers lasts for many years. The first and second drafts of the Declaration of Independence were written on paper made of hemp.

The oil of the hemp seed is reactive and prone to rancidity due to its highly unsaturated nature. Its fatty acid makeup provides a good balance of the essential fatty acids, omega-6 linoleic (55%) and omega-3 alpha-Linolenic (20%), with a ratio of 3 to 1, an especially balanced composition. Hemp oil also contains unusual and hard-to-find polyunsaturated fatty acids, gamma-Linolenic acid (GLA) at 4%, and stearidonic acid (SDA) 2%, C18:4. GLA is anti-inflammatory and supports the immune system, while the SDA is effective against atopic dermatitis and difficult skin conditions. With its broad range of fatty acids, hemp seed oil has the reputation of being called "nature's most perfectly balanced oil." Its use on the skin soothes and heals dry skin and minor burns, replenishes moisture, and protects against cellular damage.

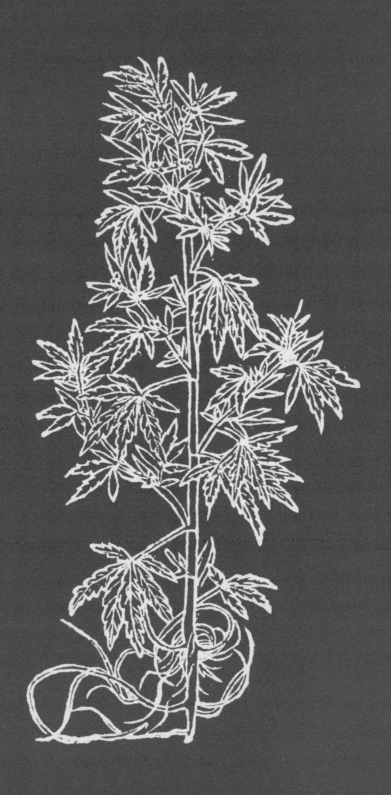

INCI — *Cannabis sativa (Hemp) Seed Oil*

Illipe butter, *Shorea stenoptera*, is extracted from the seeds of shorea, a tropical tree growing in the forests of Borneo. Traditional use in medicine, food, and skin care makes the tree an important botanical in its native region. The seed consists of 50% solid fat, which is pale yellow and turns green quickly when extracted. When refined, it becomes a solid white fat that can be used interchangeably with cocoa butter, as the triglyceride composition is similar. Soothing, non-drying, and emollient, illipe butter reinforces the skin lipid barrier function, keeping the skin moisturized.

INCI — *Shorea stenoptera (Illipe) Seed Butter*

INCI Soap — *Sodium Illipe Butterate*

Jojoba oil (ho-ho-ba), *Simmondsia chinensis*, is not technically an oil, but a liquid wax ester. Jojoba contains few triglycerides—the definition of an oil. Composed of esters and long-chain fatty acids, long carbon chains are combined with a double bond and a fatty alcohol. It looks and acts like a liquid oil, but behaves as a wax. In cold weather, it will solidify.

Jojoba was originally developed in the 1970s as a commercial product to replace sperm whale oil. A few visionaries promoted "Save the Whale" campaigns to replace sperm whale products with an environmentally sound land-based substitute. Jojoba was successfully developed as an agricultural crop, and its various products are chemically similar and even functionally superior to the "oil" from the sperm whale.

In its native Southwest and northern Mexico, jojoba nuts are eaten, and indigenous peoples have used the extracts for treating skin conditions, sores, cuts, bruises, and burns, as well as for hair care. Jojoba grows in semi-desert

⦉ **Hemp**

areas, in an environment where heat and dryness would kill most plants. The oil, or liquid wax, protects the plant by sealing the *stomata*, or pores, against evaporation in the high daytime temperatures and providing insulation against low nighttime conditions. Classed with the xerophytes, drought-resistant plants, the "oil" of Jojoba has an exceptional ability to control water loss, one of the primary causes of skin aging.

Jojoba is an excellent oil for the skin, emollient, regenerative, restructuring, and toning. It provides a light film that maintains moisture yet allows the skin to breathe. The same waxy esters are present in both jojoba and the sebum, thus its high compatibility with the skin. Miscible (capable of mixing easily with other substances without separation), it dissolves easily with the oils of the skin. Jojoba treatments lay down a non-greasy film that attracts moisture, while regulating the flow of sebum from the sebaceous glands. Jojoba, being noncomedogenic, doesn't clog pores, and protects against and treats conditions of acne. It also assists in the healthy production of the acid mantle that guards against harmful bacteria and skin imbalances. As a liquid wax, Jojoba resists oxidation and rancidity even under harsh conditions.

INCI— *Simmondsia chinensis (Jojoba) Seed Oil*

Jojoba Butter *(ho-ho-ba),* Simmondsia chinensis, has properties similar to jojoba oil. The waxy esters are made into a thick butter-like substance, even a solid wax using different degrees of hydrogenation. Different methods result in butters with different melting points, including a hard wax. There are many uses for jojoba butter in natural cosmetics, as it is said to retain the beneficial properties and qualities of the liquid form.

INCI— *Simmondsia Chinensis (Jojoba) Butter*

Karanj, *Pongamia glabra, P. pinnata,* pressed from the seeds of the pongam tree of India, is said to be a cousin to neem oil, due to its similar antibacterial properties, though they are not of the same botanical family. The oil has several unusual fatty acids that contribute to its ability to positively affect the skin. Very-long-chained behenic acid (C22:0), at 5%, gadoleic (20:1) at 10%, and lignoceric (24:0) at 2%, contribute to the oil's stability and ability to condition and protect the skin from the elements.

Karanj or karanja oil, without the strong smell and potent actions of neem, treats similar conditions. Milder and more gentle, insecticidal and antiseptic, it is used for a range of skin conditions including eczema, psoriasis, skin ulcers, dandruff, and to promote wound healing. A traditional herb plant, all its parts, leaves, seeds, and bark have been used for centuries in northern India. As a treatment for parasites and as an antidote for poisoning, it is a native herbal pharmacy. Karanj oil can be made into soap and used on the hair, used for pets with skin conditions, and used as a therapeutic skin wash.

INCI — *Pongamia Glabra (Karanja) Seed Oil*

Kiwi fruit seed oil, *Actinidia chinesis,* is a plant indigenous to the island country of New Zealand. Kiwi seed oil consists of majority omega-3 fatty acids, which produce anti-inflammatory metabolites that are soothing to the skin. Uncommonly high in the essential fatty acids alpha-Linolenic (60%) and linoleic (20%), it is one of the richest sources of these nutrients for the skin and body. Its 3:1 omega-3 to 6 ratio makes it an oil that can be used for treating and balancing inflammatory conditions.

Kiwi fruit seed oil is non-oily, penetrating the skin easily, and with a low viscosity it has a light comfortable feel. The phospholipid content can be observed in a light whitish film that develops when the oil is applied to wet skin. Highly nutritious, kiwi is one of the oils high in natural vitamin C. When the vitamin is delivered naturally, it benefits the skin tissues without danger of oxidation or irritation. Nutrients in kiwi seed oil, including fatty acid properties, vitamins C and E, potassium, and magnesium, help in repairing sun damage, while nourishing and regenerating the skin layers. The oil absorbs easily, is readily taken up by the tissues, and is pleasant to work with.

INCI— *Actinidia chinesis (Kiwi) Seed Oil*

Kukui nut oil, *Aleurtes moluccana*, is a non-edible oil belonging
to the same botanical family as the castor bean plant, *Euphorbia*. Neither oil is used for food, as they cause gastric distress when ingested. Kukui is the state tree of Hawaii and was brought to the islands by the early Polynesian settlers. In Hawaii the common name for kukui is candlenut, as the ancient Hawaiians used the nuts for light, burning them on stone lamps or stringing and lighting them. In old Hawaii, kukui nut oil was used for skin care, particularly for protecting newborn infants and children from the sun, salt, and weather.

Kukui nut oil, high in the essential fatty acids, alpha-Linolenic acid (30%) and linoleic acid (40%), has a similar lipid composition to the oils of the skin. Kukui oil is thus easily incorporated into the stratum corneum, due to the essential fatty acids and oleic acid (30%). Strengthening the intracellular bonds that support the structure of the skin, the oil lays down a mixture of saturated (16%) and unsaturated fatty acids, leaving a semi-permeable layer that nourishes, protects, and prevents premature aging. Containing vitamins A, C, and E, the oil is anti-inflammatory and aids circulation while helping alleviate skin problems such as eczema, psoriasis, and rosacea. It is useful in treating people with difficult skin conditions and for wounds, as it prevents scarring. For use on infants and children, it is protective and moisturizing to their delicate skin.

INCI — *Aleurtes moluccana (Kukui Nut) Seed Oil*

INCI Soap — *Sodium Kukuiate*

Macadamia nut oil, *Macadamia ternifolia*, is also known as *Queensland nut oil* in its original home, Australia. Macadamia trees were imported to the Hawaiian islands in 1882, where they have since become an important and valuable crop. The oil is used for cooking and for skin care products, and the nuts are delicious dipped in chocolate, a favorite in the islands!

Macadamia nut oil has emollient properties, with a high (up to 60%) monounsaturated oleic acid content. More importantly, it is one of the few vegetable oils high in palmitoleic acid (at 20%), which is a building block lipid of the skin. Significant quantities of the fatty acid are rare in vegetable oils, as it is more often found in fish oils. Palmitoleic acid acts as an anti-microbial agent, protecting against cellular breakdown in wounds and skin abrasions. As an antioxidant, it protects cell lipids from UV damage from oxidation. When young, our skin contains palmitoleic acid, but the level decreases with age. Supplementation with macadamia nut oil is one means of protecting the skin in later years.

Macadamia nut oil, with its important range of fatty acids, supports cellular membranes, nourishes the skin, and provides a lipid barrier to retain moisture and regenerate the skin layers. Its squalene content supplements the amount found in the stratum corneum, helping to regenerate skin cells and protect against chapping and weather damage. Macadamia nut oil provides hydrating and gentle care for mature skin, and is recommended for lip care. The unrefined oil can be strongly scented of nuts, something that needs to be considered when developing products.

INCI— *Macadamia ternifolia (Macadamia Nut) Seed Oil*

Soap—*Sodium Macadamiate*

Maize oil—see **Corn oil**

Mango butter, *Mangifera indica,* comes from a native tree of India. The butter is pressed from the large seed kernel of the fruit. ("Butter" is a term often used to describe saturated oils that are solid at room temperature.) High amounts (up to 5%) of nutritive unsaponifiable plant compounds give mango butter rejuvenating and wound-healing properties as well as UV ray-protective capabilities. The caffeic acid present in the butter is also a particularly powerful antioxidant and fungicide. Mangiferin, a polyphenol specific to mango, provides antioxidant, anti-fungal, and anti-inflammatory properties. Tannins in the oil create a dry-feeling butter, providing astringency with a light feel on the skin.

As one of the oils containing a fair amount of natural and stable vitamin C, along with saturated and unsaturated fatty acid content, mango butter is able to moisturize, repair, and revitalize the skin layers. Mango butter gives salves a wonderful soft texture when used with other unsaturated oils and beeswax. In soap or cosmetic formulas, it is used as an active principle that supports and nourishes the skin.

INCI— *Mangifera indica (Mango Butter) Seed Oil*

INCI Soap—*Sodium Mango Butterate*

Maracuja, see **Passion fruit seed oil**

Marula oil, *Sclerocarya birrea*, is another botanical contribution

from Africa now gaining popularity in the West for skin care. Called "miracle oil," marula is considered one of Africa's botanical treasures. The oil has an extensive and deep presence in western and southern Africa. Belonging to the same botanical family as the mango, it is used for cooking, preserving meat, body care, and infant care.

Marula oil, very high in oleic acid (70%), with some linoleic acid (6%), and saturated palmitic acid (10%), improves the ability of the skin to hold moisture deep in its layers. A small amount of the very-long-chain erucic fatty acid gives the oil a feeling of substance and body. Softening and soothing the complexion, marula absorbs well and has a silky feel when used for massage and body conditioning. Rich in antioxidants, the oil has impressive oxidative stability, helping to extend the shelf life of products made with it due to its high levels of polyphenols, vitamin C, and E.

The flavonoids, procyanidins, proanthocyanidins, gallotannins, and catechins also work as antioxidants on the skin, providing healing and anti-inflammatory properties. Phytosterols help improve the skin's ability to retain moisture by protecting the barrier function of the stratum corneum. A noticeable phospholipid content is particularly nourishing for cell walls and helps with skin absorption and emulsification.

INCI — *Sclerocarya birrea (Marula) oil*

Meadowfoam seed oil, *Limnanthes alba,* was developed as

an agricultural crop in the 1970s as an alternative to sperm whale oil. In this regard it has a history similar to jojoba in the Southwest. A native wildflower of the northwestern United States, its name expresses the way a field of the crop appears when in bloom, like white foam blowing across the sea.

A distinctive oil, the majority (97%) of meadowfoam's fatty acid composition is 20 carbons long or longer—highly unusual in a vegetable oil.

The fatty acid composition is what gives the oil its extraordinary stability and with a high percentage of vitamin E, meadowfoam actually helps to preserve products to which it is added. Liquid at room temperature and of a high molecular weight, it feels thick but not greasy. The oil adheres to the skin and protects it. The composition of the oil makes it particularly protective and rejuvenating to the skin. Possessing sun-screening properties, it is increasingly used in products for sun protection. The ability to moisturize and protect skin and hair, along with its durable shelf life, makes meadowfoam seed oil a valued addition to the product-makers' options.

INCI—*Limnanthes alba oil*

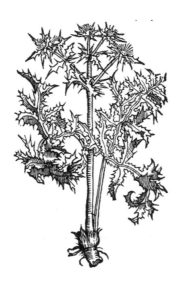

Milk thistle seed oil, *Silybum marianum*, is an oil pressed from the seeds of the important liver herb. The oil is a by-product of the extraction of silymarin, a hepatoprotective active ingredient used to treat liver failure and poisoning. Silymarin's flavonoid properties protect and regenerate damaged cells and can detoxify and restore the liver to normal functioning. Silymarin has been used successfully in cases of cirrhosis, mushroom poisoning, and hepatitis. By protecting the liver from the side effects of medical treatments like chemotherapy, silymarin can help strengthen the body while it heals. Silymarin is a flavonoid complex, an antioxidant, and a membrane-stabilizing compound. The oil retains some measure of the compound, and how much depends on the extraction and refining process used.

Milk thistle oil also contains polyunsaturated fatty acids, mainly linoleic acid, at up to 65%. The plant healing fractions are abundant, with phytosterols including beta-sitosterol, stigmasterol, and campesterol, as well as phospholipids and squalene. The seeds and oil are high in vitamin E and antioxidants that nourish and repair damage to the skin and body. Skin cells are hydrated and deeply supplied with compounds for repair and regeneration.

INCI — *Silybum marianum (Milk Thistle) Seed Oil*

Moringa oil, *Moringa oleifera*, has been found in Egyptian burial

tombs. The leaves, nuts, and oil of moringa were used by the ancient Egyptians as food and skin care, and were an important part of Egyptian culture. An African name for the tree is *nebeday*, which means "the tree that never dies," a reference to its longevity, and "miracle tree," for the highly nutritious compounds and beneficial properties it provides.

The oil is commercially known as *Ben oil* or *Behen oil*, due to its relatively high content of behenic acid (10%). The very-long-chained saturated fatty acid (C22:0) helps the oil resist rancidity for up to five years. In perfumery, the oil is used in a technique called enfleurage, the process of extracting scents from delicate flowers by transferring the compounds to a fat or oil. The very-long-chain fatty acids extract and help to hold the most delicate and fugitive scents in perfumery.

Rich in monounsaturated oleic acid (70%), the oil is emollient and moisturizing, able to heal roughness and dry skin. With its behenic acid content, moringa oil is less oily than many oils high in oleic acid, a property esteemed in the cosmetics industry. Very high anti-oxidative properties contribute to moringa's stability while protecting skin and hair from damage by oxidation or environment.

INCI: *Moringa Oleifera Seed Oil*

Neem oil, *Azadirachta indica,* from the plant native to India, can be

considered one of the original medicines, having been in use for over 4,000 years. Now grown across the semi-tropics it is used as a local "pharmacy" in villages and towns. All parts of the tree are used, including the leaves and twigs for tea, and the seeds for oil and meal. The oil of neem is antibacterial, antiviral, anti-fungal, antiseptic, and anti-parasitic. Very strong-smelling, neem oil is semi-solid at room temperature.

Neem oil can be used topically, although it should be diluted with another oil to avoid irritation. Some suppliers dilute the oil before sale, so check the percentage before purchasing. Dilutions from 2% to 50%, depending on applications, are recommended. Generally, higher dilutions are suggested when used directly on the skin. The properties in the oil are so strong that many conditions require only a few drops added to a shampoo, soap, or oil. The oil should only be used internally under the guidance of a qualified health care professional familiar with its actions. Internal use of neem oil is strong medicine, and can cause health problems if not used properly.

Topically, neem can treat athlete's foot and fungal conditions, kill bacteria when used in soap and salves, and can be used as an insect repellent. Neem contains vitamin E and essential fatty acids that moisturize and regenerate the cells of the skin. As one of the most active fixed oils, neem is a valuable healer and invites respect.

INCI— *Azadirachta indica (Neem) Seed Oil*

INCI Soap— *Sodium Neemate*

Nigella/Black seed oil, *Nigella sativa*, from the buttercup family, *Ranunculaceae*, has been a staple of the Mediterranean and Arabic cultures since antiquity. The tiny black nigella seed has a number of popular names and is known as black cumin seed, black caraway, onion seed, and coriander seed, though it has no relation to the spice cumin or caraway, onions or coriander. The taste and smell are strong and a bit peppery. Try a teaspoon of the oil in fresh orange juice for a delicious EFA supplement.

The seeds have been used for food, oil, and medicine for thousands of years. Seeds found in Tutankhamen's tomb signify both nigella's antiquity and its importance in Egyptian culture, as only items and foods that would assist the pharaoh in the afterlife were placed in his tomb. The earliest written account of black seed is in the Old Testament book of Isaiah, where the prophet contrasts the importance of black seed with that of wheat.

Mohamed is said to have declared black seed the remedy for "every disease except death." Modern analysis of the seed and oil supports the validity of his enthusiasm. The seeds are packed with over one hundred identified nutrients. The essential fatty acids, linoleic acid (58%), and alpha-Linolenic acid (0.2%), zinc, calcium, folacin, iron, copper, phosphorus, riboflavin, thiamin, pyridoxine, carotenes, protein, carbohydrate, fiber, and a number of polyunsaturated fatty acids are found in the ground meal.

Nigella's use as a medicine includes topical treatment of psoriasis, eczema, sore joints, and dry skin. As an internal remedy, it is used for treating headaches, nasal congestion, intestinal worms, liver, and digestive disorders. With its ability to also support the immune system, it has a well-deserved reputation.

INCI — *Nigella sativa Seed Oil*

Oat seed oil, *Avena sativa,* is a luxurious oil from the common oat

grain. Highly emollient and rich, the oil soothes and conditions the skin. Oats are classed as nervines (nervous system tonics) in western herbalism for their ability to soothe and calm jagged nerves and conditions. A very finely ground form of oat flour called colloidal oat is approved by the FDA as a treatment for dry and itchy skin. It is a popular external treatment for irritated and itchy skin conditions. The oil shares similar properties as the dry and fresh herb, and the actions are helpful for calming and repairing damaged, sensitive, and tender skin.

With a balanced ratio of oleic and linoleic acid of about 40% each, oat oil is particularly beneficial for the stratum corneum. The saturated palmitic acid, with its relatively short carbon chain, soothes and protects the outer skin layer. Rich in vitamin E complex, antioxidants, and carotenoids, oat oil is a strong yellow color and deeply emollient. Over twenty unique polyphenols specific to oats are anti-inflammatory, anti-proliferative, and anti-itching. Of particular interest are avenanthramides, strong antioxidants produced by the plant as a defense against fungal invasion. Beta-glucan, a rich source of polysaccharides and soluble fiber, along with phospholipids, aids emulsification, to make oat oil a skin-soothing addition to skin creams and compounded products. The oil is fairly new on the market as a cosmetic ingredient, but interest in its unique qualities and applications is beginning to grow.

INCI — *Avena sativa (Oat) Seed Oil*

Nigella. Raden.

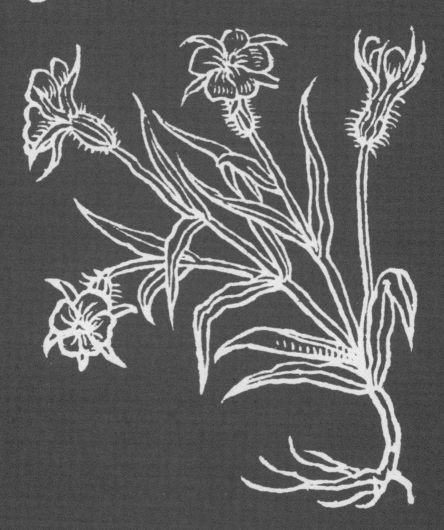

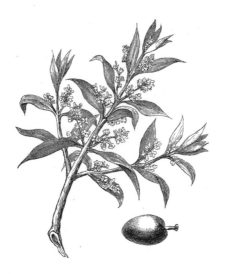

Olive oil, *Olea europaea,* from a member of the family containing lilacs, jasmine, and the ash tree *Oleaceae,* is another of the ancient food and oil crops. In the historical Middle East, olive trees were extremely valuable and the oil used as a form of currency. So important was the crop the word "oil" in Greek, is the same as "olive." "Offering an olive branch" is the accepted gesture for peace. And it was an olive branch that the dove brought back to Noah on the ark, signaling the end of the flood. In Greek myth, Athena threw her javelin into the air, and where it landed the first olive tree burst forth. Athens was named in her honor for the gift of precious oil and food she provided. Olive trees are long-lived and there are specimens in Israel said to be over a thousand years old.

Stories of anointing oils are told throughout the Bible. In anointing animals, sanctuaries, wafers, stones, heads of men and women, and even kings, the oil of olives was used to bless people and sanctify objects in many stories. As a significant oil in human history, it is fitting that the very common and abundant fatty acid oleic acid is named for the olive and makes up a large percentage of the oil, around 70%.

Olive is a stable oil, able to tolerate some heat and exposure to light. In skin care, oleic acid supports the natural breathing process and sebum production of the skin. Phytosterols provide humectant properties, attracting moisture to the skin and aiding in the repair of sun-damaged tissues while moisturizing and soothing very dry skin.

Olive oil is a major source of plant-based squalene, one of the most common lipids produced by skin cells. As a natural part of sebum, squalene lubricates the skin, prevents the evaporation of moisture, and functions as a natural emollient and protective agent. Found in rice bran oil as well as olive, squalene supports the delivery of oxygen to skin cells and removes waste. A deficiency of squalene results in dry skin and premature aging. Said to have a molecular structure similar to vitamin A, squalene is highly unsaturated and valuable for skin health. As a precursor of phytosterols, squalene was first discovered in a pure form in shark livers. Vegetable-sourced squalene is extracted from the olive and other vegetable sources.

INCI — *Olea europaea (Olive) Fruit Oil*

Olive is a choice oil for soap, with its beneficial effect on the skin, relatively low cost, and wide availability. For centuries, castile soaps were made with 100% olive oil. Cold process soaps of pure olive oil make a lovely bar that has a soft feel but produces little lather. As an unsaturated oil, olive oil saponifies slowly, but in combination with saturated oils it makes lovely soap with skin-conditioning properties.

INCI Soap — *Sodium Olivate*

Olive/Pomace oil, *Olea europaea,* is the oil pressed from the
hard pits, the pomace, of olives after the virgin oil has been pressed from the fruit. It is an inferior grade of olive oil for cooking, but is inexpensive and

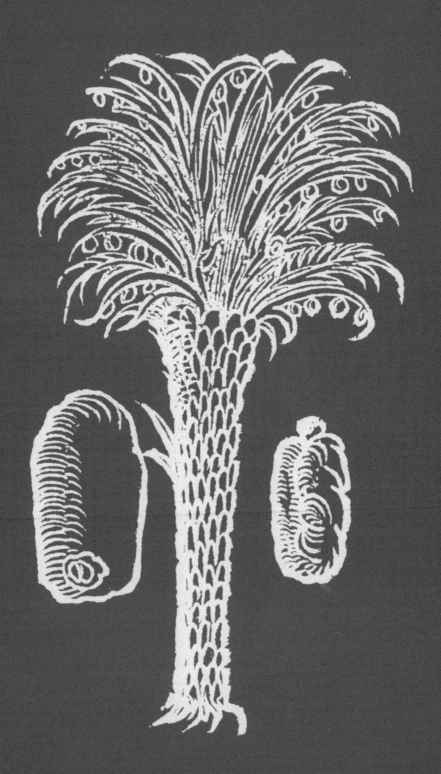

useful for making soap. Pomace oil's high unsaponifiable content creates a thick, viscous mix that reacts quickly, bringing all the oils into saponification.

INCI — *Olea europaea (Olive) Seed Oil*

INCI Soap — *Sodium Olivate*

Ootanga oil, see **Watermelon seed oil**

Palm oil, *Elaeis guineensis*, is pressed from the pulp of the fruit of the African oil palm and is the source for the fatty acid names palmitic and palmitoleic. It is a member of the same family, *Arecaceae,* as coconut, babassu, and acai, all of which are palms. The pulp is a naturally strong red-orange. When this fleshy or fibrous part around the kernel, the mesocarp, is pressed, a solid red-orange oil is the result. Highly colored with natural beta-carotene, palm oil is used for cooking and skin care in its native Africa. In the West, Middle Eastern markets and more recently local co-ops carry the red version of the oil for cooking. An excellent source of pro-vitamin A carotenoids, it turns food a deep golden color. The pale yellow version of palm oil is refined of color and available from oil suppliers for making soap and cosmetics.

Palm oil's unsaponifiable compounds are naturally rich in carotenoids, as evidenced by the red color. These are precursors of vitamin A, a nutrient that promotes cell regeneration. The beta and other carotenes are abundant in the unrefined red oil, but less so in the pale refined version. Palm oil's primarily saturated fatty acids reinforce, support, and protect the cutaneous layer of the skin.

Since the original edition of this study in 2001, palm oil has become linked to habitat destruction in tropical countries. Finding sustainably farmed sources of palm oil is important. Habitats and whole ecological environments

⟨ **Palm**

have been destroyed to support demands from other parts of the world for oil. Wild areas need our protection so that we do not lose what they have so freely and generously provided.

INCI — *Elaeis guineensis (Palm) Oil*

Soap made exclusively with palm oil is brittle and drying on the skin. But when combined with coconut and unsaturated oils, its high percentage of saturated fatty acids adds hardness and longevity to the final soap. Palm oils are less water-soluble than other oils, saponifying easily due to its saturated state, and the resulting hard bars of soap have staying power.

INCI Soap — *Sodium Palmate*

Palm Kernel oil, *Elaeis guineensis*, is also pressed from the African oil palm but from the kernels, not the pulp and fruit. Palm kernel oil is a pale cream to white color, distinctly different from the fruit's red oil. It is also very hard at room temperature, having a higher saturated fatty acid profile than palm fruit oil. The large proportion of lauric acid, almost 50% in the kernel, provides both saturation and low molecular weight, characteristics that produce hard bars soaps. The low molecular weight of the lauric acid in both coconut and palm kernel oils produces lather that is easy and full in all kinds of water.

INCI — *Elaeis guineensis (Palm kernel) Oil*

INCI Soap — *Sodium Palm Kernelate*

Papaya seed oil, *Carica papaya*, is from the seeds of the tropical fruit. Papaya seed oil is included for a dear relative who lived in Hawaii years ago, and grew papaya fruit on tall skinny trees in the backyard. She once mailed me papaya seeds, quite illegally breaking many agricultural import/export

regulations, and asking if I could make something with them in my workshop. She hated to see them go to waste and would supply them abundantly. At the time, there was no such thing as papaya seed oil, nor did I have a press to make it had I even considered the possibility. The amazing thing about botanical oils in the twenty-first century is our ability to extract the fatty acids from more and more sources and transport them all over the world. Now, years later, we do have papaya seed oil. A testament to her foresight.

Sometimes called the paw paw tree or fruit, papaya is a tropical herbaceous tree that is killed by frost. When trees are young they produce fruit within reach, but as they grow taller and taller each year, the fruit is soon unattainable. Eventually the trees are blown over in storms or high winds. Papaya fruit and oil contain an enzyme, papain, that clears the skin of debris and dead cells, making it an ideal oil for exfoliating masks and treatments. Said to remove or fade dark skin spots, it is an oil useful in caring for mature skin. High in oleic acid (70%), and palmitic acid (16%), the oil is quite stable. Used as a massage oil, it is rejuvenating to the skin, with antibacterial properties that enhance wound healing and skin-repair functions. With minerals, vitamins A and C, and amino acids, papaya seed oil is nourishing and strengthens the tissues. Anti-inflammatory properties soothe soreness and muscle cramps.

INCI — *Carica papaya (Papaya) Seed Oil*

Passion fruit seed oil, *Passiflora incarnata,* is also called

maracuja oil or *passion flower oil*. The passion vine, a native of the Amazon basin, grows from tropical to temperate regions in North and South America. Producing an exquisite flower, the vine reaches up to 150 feet. The yellow fruit and pink flesh is sweet and juicy but full of seeds. In Hawaii, passion fruit is called lilikoi and made into juice and jams. The high vitamin C content of the fruit is also present in the oil, helping support collagen formation in the skin. Massaged on the skin, the oil feels soft and soothing, relaxing tissues and calming the body. It is a full-bodied oil that helps relax tissues before sinking into the skin.

The plant and flower are used in herbal preparations for calming the nervous system, relieving stress, and for sleep disorders. Passion fruit oil contains calcium and phosphorous, minerals that support a healthy nervous system with the ability to soothe and calm nerves. With anti-inflammatory, anti-spasmodic, and sedative properties, the oil is good for use in massage, baby care, and skin care. Its high linoleic acid content (77%) makes it light and easily absorbed. Passion fruit seed oil benefits aging, dry, and cracked skin and other difficult skin conditions.

INCI— *Passiflora incarnata (Passion fruit) Seed Oil*

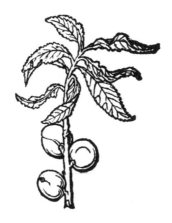

Peach kernel oil, *Prunus persica,* is from a tree with origins in China. The oil is pressed from the kernels of the fruit. As with other oils from members of the rose family (such as apricot, almond, plum, and cherry), peach kernel oil is emollient, moisturizing, protective, and nourishing. Peach kernels are high in boron, a trace nutrient necessary for maintaining bone and joint health. The health of the skin is improved by the high content of vitamins

E and A, as well as some B vitamins. Predominantly composed of oleic (60%) and linoleic acid (30%), the oil leaves skin protected and nourished. The feel of the oil on the skin is very light, penetrating, silky, and smooth. Peach kernel oil benefits anti-aging treatments and helps dry and sensitive skin. It is also usually well-tolerated by sensitive individuals, and some have found it to be hypo-allergenic for those with allergies to nut oils like peanut.

INCI— *Prunus persica (Peach) Kernel Oil*

INCI Soap— *Sodium Peach Kernelate*

Pecan oil, *Algooquian pacaan,* or *Carya pecan,* is primarily an oil for cooking, but can be used for soap and body care. 50% oleic acid and 40% linoleic acid, it has properties that are beneficial for a variety of skin care uses. Being of the *Juglandaceae* family, its cousins walnut and hickory have similar properties. A light oil with little to no scent or color, it has a relatively short shelf life, between six months and a year.

INCI— *Algooquian pacaan (Pecan) Nut Oil*

Peanut oil, *Arachis hypogeae,* is a useful soap-making oil due to its low cost and easy availability. Usually found in bulk in Asian food markets or obtained from their suppliers, it contains high amounts of vitamin E and is easily absorbed by the skin. The oil, about 50% oleic acid and 35% percent linoleic, also contains the very-long-chain saturated fatty acids behenic acid (22:0) at 3% and lignoceric acid (24:0) at about 1%. These very-long-chain fatty acids give the oil body, and a good feel for use in skin care and massage. In soap, peanut oil provides a lather that is thin but long-lasting. *Note:* peanuts are an allergen for sensitive people, both internally and externally. This oil is best used cautiously, and label products clearly.

INCI — *Arachis hypogeae (Peanut) Oil*

INCI Soap — *Sodium Peanutate*

Pequi oil, *Caryocar braziliensis,* comes from a tree native to Brazil. The nuts are eaten and the oil is a valuable part of the culture, used for food preparation, skin, and hair care by the native population. The predominant fatty acid profile is a balance of oleic and palmitic acids, which are protective with monounsaturated and saturated properties. Minor amounts of additional skin-beneficial fatty acids, including palmitoleic, alpha-Linolenic, myristic, and linoleic, make the oil well-balanced and conditioning for mature skin care. Pequi oil is high in vitamins E and A, and nourishing as a moisturizer. Often promoted for hair care, it is able to smooth the cuticle of the hair, protecting it from dryness and preventing frizziness. With antioxidants quercetin and gallic acid, the oil is anti-inflammatory, anti-fungal, and anti-microbial, which makes it helpful in working with conditions of eczema, psoriasis, and cracked dry skin.

INCI — *Caryocar braziliensis (Pequi) Seed Oil*

Perilla seed oil, *Perilla frutescens,* comes from an herb grown and used extensively in China, Japan, and other Asian cultures. In Japan, its common names are *beefsteak plant* or *shiso.* Perilla, a member of the mint or *Laminaceae* family and grown as an annual, has leaves that can be green or red. The red-leaved variety is used to color and pickle foods. In Japan, umeboshi (salt plums) are made red by shiso leaves and ginger slices are pickled and colored pink when mixed with the leaves. The leaves contain anti-microbial and preserving properties, which is why they are used to pickle foods.

Oil from the seeds of perilla is very high in essential fatty acids, especially the omega-3 alpha-Linolenic acid (as high as 65%), rivaling flax seed oil. Balanced with linoleic acid (10 to 20%), it is classed as a drying oil and has been used for making paint, varnish, inks, lacquers, and flooring in Asia. Its high alpha-Linolenic acid content makes perilla oil unstable, and if purchased in bulk, it needs to be kept refrigerated and used quickly.

Perilla's antiseptic and antimicrobial properties from rosmarinic acid make it useful in treatments for acne and difficult skin conditions. The high content of essential fatty acids nourishes and helps retain moisture, protecting the health of the stratum corneum. Absorbing rapidly, perilla seed oil conditions, and its unusual and beneficial properties help treat skin problems such as eczema and psoriasis.

INCI— *Perilla frutescens (Perilla) Seed Oil*

Pistachio nut oil, *Pistacia vera,* is a native of the Middle East
and an integral part of regional cooking traditions. It is highly unsaturated, with a high level of essential fatty acids, especially linoleic acid (up to 35%) and monounsaturated oleic acid (at 50%). Pistachio nut oil is non-greasy and absorbed easily by the skin, moisturizing and softening, limiting water loss. Pistachio nut oil provides a dry emollience and is noncomedogenic, preventing oil build-up on the skin. It has natural resistance to oxidation and rancidity, due to highly antioxidant compounds in the nuts that help to prolong shelf life of products. Pistachio oil is a good skin care oil.

INCI— *Pistacia vera (Pistachio) Nut Oil*

Plum kernel oil, *Prunus domestica,* is another from the rose
family of plants. The oil is pressed from the pits of the fruit and is highly scented of bitter almonds or marzipan. With many of the same attributes

of the other rose family oils, such as peach, cherry, almond and apricot, it is high in oleic acid, with linoleic and palmitic in lesser quantities. Excellent for skin care, with generous amounts of vitamin E, it also provides small amounts of a variety of the trace very-long-chain fatty acids so necessary for skin health.

INCI— *Prunus domestica (Plum) Seed Oil*

Pomegranate seed oil, *Punica granatum,* is a rich and

elegant oil containing unique punicic acid (C18:3) at 75%. Punicic fatty acid is named for the pomegranate, *Punica*, in which it was found. The plant, native to areas of Iran through northern India, has been cultivated across the Mediterranean since ancient times. Nearly exclusive to pomegranate and found in the oils of two gourd seeds, punicic acid is a highly nutritious fatty acid for the skin, able to balance pH and condition the skin's surface. The fatty acid is anti-inflammatory, anti-microbial, and cell regenerating, helping to increase elasticity of the skin and repair sun and weather damage.

Punicic acid is an omega-5 fatty acid and its long-chain, superunsaturated fatty acids with three conjugated double bonds are an unusual form. The conjugated double bonds cause the oil to feel thick and rich on the skin, delivering the oil's beneficial properties effectively to the tissues.

Possessing a variety of phytohormones, phytosterols, flavonoids, and polyphenols, the anti-oxidative properties deeply penetrate and protect against free radical damage in the skin tissues. Gallic acid heals wounds and soothes burns, while ellagic acid protects and rebuilds collagen and provides added thickness to thin skin. Anti-inflammatory and regenerative, the oil is of particular benefit for mature complexions, supporting collagen production and providing protection from environmental exposure. Researchers have conducted studies of pomegranate seed oil on cancer tissues, breast tissues in particular, with promising results. A pale color, pomegranate seed oil has little scent but a luxurious feel on the skin.

INCI—*Punica granatum (Pomegrante) Seed oil*

Poppy seed oil, *Papaver somniferum*, is obtained by pressing the

seeds of the opium poppy flower. Potent alkaloids, found in the pods, flowers, and somewhat in the stems, are absent in the seed, which contains only a trace if any amount. Poppy seed oil has culinary, pharmaceutical, and even industrial uses, where it is made into paints, varnishes, and soaps. It is a palatable oil that had wider acceptance as food in the past. Now it is used more often in industry and medicine. As a painting medium, it is clear and doesn't yellow.

The oil, a rich source of linoleic acid (70%) and oleic acid (16%), is colorless and has very little scent. Poppy seed is considered to have good moisturizing properties, and can be used to make a wide variety of cosmetic products. The oil is absorbed by the skin deeply and easily. It contains properties similar to hemp seed, and can be used as a substitute. Similarly, it needs refrigeration in storage to protect it from oxidation.

INCI—*Papaver somniferum (Poppy) Seed oil*

Pracaxi oil, *Pentaclethara macroloba*, is a native of tropical wet

areas of South America. Named *pracaxi* by the Portuguese, in Brazil it is simply "*oil tree*." Pracaxi oil, pressed from the seeds and fruit, is unusual in that it has one of the highest concentrations of behenic acid (C22:0), 10 to 25%, similar to but higher than moringa. Behenic acid is a saturated fatty acid that is poorly absorbed by the body when ingested, but adds protective properties to oils when used externally. Peanuts and rapeseed are other rich sources of the fatty acid. Having a very long chain, as well as being saturated, this fatty acid lends great stability to oils containing it.

The skin feel of pracaxi is heavy, almost waxy, coating the skin with a feeling of thick oil. Externally, small amounts of pracaxi oil are especially beneficial as a hair conditioner, where it has a reputation for disentangling and brightening. The oil is solid at room temperature in the temperate zone, yet melts on contact with the skin. With oleic acid (55%), and linoleic acid (20%), it is emollient and protective. In its native Amazon basin, pracaxi is used as an insect repellent, for stretch marks, to brighten the skin, and minimize scarring. Medicinally, drugs are made with it for use against snakebite and hemorrhagic conditions.

INCI — *Pentaclethara macroloba (Pracaxi) Seed oil*

Pumpkin seed oil, *Cucurbita pepo,* has a long history used as a

food oil rather than for topical applications. It is dark in color with a strong nutty flavor, very thick, and looks a bit like motor oil, but has a nut-like scent. Styrian pumpkin seeds, native to Styria (a region of southeastern Austria), grow without an outer shell, making oil processing easy. Traditionally, the seeds are lightly roasted before pressing, although raw seed oils can be found.

The oil has an extensive background in medicine and food, and is high in essential fatty acids, especially linoleic acid (55%). It is also high in vitamins and minerals, especially zinc, copper, and manganese. Caffeic acid and tocopherols act as free radical scavengers, protecting against oxidation and cell damage. High in carotenoids, precursors of vitamin A, the oil helps reduce redness and itching, acting as an anti-inflammatory. Phytosterols provide moisturizing and protective properties to the skin. Traditional uses of pumpkin seed oil are in food and cooking. For the skin, it provides high levels of polyunsaturated fatty acids and nourishing compounds. The color

Pumpkin ⟩

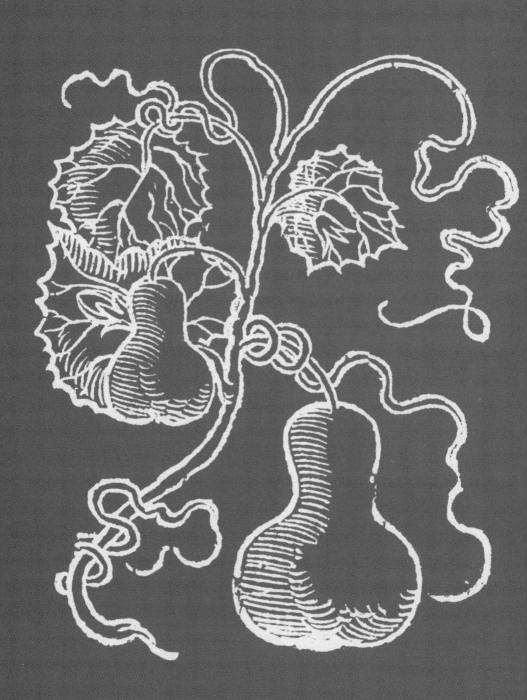

and scent, however, are strong and not always welcome in skin care products.

INCI — *Cucurbita pepo (Pumpkin) Seed Oil*

Red raspberry seed oil, Rubus idaeus, is a specialty oil and by-

product of raspberry juice production. The oil from the seeds can be found cold pressed or hexane-extracted. With high concentrations of essential fatty acids, including omega-3 at 25%, and 52% omega-6, it has an oxidative stability greater than its fatty acid makeup suggests. The long shelf life is due to a high antioxidant and phospholipid content, making the oil excellent for skin conditioning.

Exceptionally high in vitamins E and provitamin A, the oil has been identified as having potential for sun protection. The plant compounds in raspberry seed oil are being studied for use as a broad spectrum UV-A and UV-B sunscreen. Claims are being made for a potential SPF of somewhere between 28 and 50 when the oil is used without dilution on the skin. An SPF that high is comparable to titanium dioxide and would be exceptional in an oil, should the studies be confirmed. Raspberry oil is exceptionally light, and sinks into the surface of the skin quickly, creating a dry but moisturized feel. The oil has a slight raspberry scent and feels like summer any time of year.

INCI — *Rubus Idaeus (Raspberry) Seed Oil*

Rice bran oil, Oryza sativa, is pressed from the germ and pericarp of

the rice seed, which contains from 16 to 20% oil. It is rich in unsaponifiable elements, at 4%. Phytosterols including gamma-oryzanol and ferulic acid, when combined, become a potent antioxidant for cell membranes in animals and humans. Rice bran oil is also a source of vegetable-based squalene, an important element of our skin's lipid production. Functioning as an antioxidant, squalene helps guard against age spots, stopping the oxidation process in the skin. Squalene is also a vital part of the production of sterols in both plants and animals, and that includes the synthesis of vitamin D in the skin of humans.

The ferulic acid content of rice bran oil, in addition to being antioxidant, suppresses melanin generation in the skin layers. Melanin is the pigment structure in the skin that protects the cells against excess sun. In Japan, where pale and un-tanned complexions are desirable, ferulic acid extracts are popular. The compound, in oil or as an extract, absorbs harmful long-wave ultraviolet rays. This ability to interfere with free radical and active oxidative activity and to block UV rays makes rice bran oil a useful component of sunscreen treatments.

INCI — *Oryza sativa (Rice) Bran Oil*

INCI Soap — *Sodium Ricate*

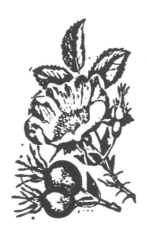

Rose hip seed oil, *Rosa rubiginosa*, is pressed from the seeds of wild Chilean rose hips, and its use by the native population extends over centuries. Regenerative and nourishing, rose hip seed oil has a number of compounds that directly benefit the skin. Its fatty acid profile is noteworthy, with nearly equal percentages of alpha-Linolenic and linoleic acid of close to 40% each. A generously endowed oil, its vitamin A content increases elastin content, promotes collagen formation, and helps to delay age-related breakdown of the skin and underlying tissues. Vitamins E and C help to delay the onset of skin aging, nourishing the cells and shielding against oxidation while creating a lipid barrier that protects and supports the skin. Tannins add astringent qualities to rose hip seed oil, giving it a dry noncomedogenic quality. Rose hip seed oil has been found in clinical trials to be active in cell regeneration and a treatment for scar tissue and blemishes. The ability of the oil to heal and maintain the texture and softness of the skin is noteworthy. Deep wrinkles, UV damage, dark spots, uneven pigmentation, and difficult skin conditions are improved by the use of rose hip seed oil.

Rose hip seed oil varies significantly in color, from pale yellow to a rich deeply golden orange color. Organic rose hip seed oils have the strongest natural color, while conventional oils are usually pale. The depth of color in the oil indicates the presence of beneficial compounds such as carotenoids and natural vitamins. Vitamin C, minerals, lycopene, and other carotenoids present in rose hip seed oil provide significant health-giving properties. On the skin, the oil has a silky and luscious feel, absorbing quickly and completely, creating a moisture barrier.

INCI—*Rosa Mosqueta (Rosehip) Fruit Oil*

Sacha inchi, *Plukenetia volubilis,* peruvian mountain peanut, sacha peanut, or inca peanut, also on occasion called pracaxi, is distinct from *Pentaclethara spp.*—a different plant all together. Sacha inchi belongs to the botanical family *Euphorbiaceae*, of which kukui and castor nuts are members. Unlike those members from the extremely large family, sacha inchi nuts and oil are said to be particularly digestible and easy on the stomach. The plant is a large climbing vine native to the rain forests of Peru, and indigenous people have cultivated and eaten the nuts and used the oil for centuries.

As one of a handful of oils with high percentages of linoleic and alpha-Linolenic fatty acids, and only minor amounts of oleic acid, sacha inchi oil is helpful for problem skin and hard-to-treat skin conditions. The nuts and oil are also suitable for omega-3 dietary supplementation and are high in proteins, vitamins A and E, and tryptophan, nourishing and helping alleviate depression and nutritional deficiencies. Rich in the phytonutrients, the oil has an impressive 18-month shelf life. It also helps with dry, itchy, scaly, and irritated skin, nourishing both internally and externally.

INCI — *Plukenetia volubilis (Sacha Inchi) Oil*

Safflower oil, *Carthamus tinctorius*, comes from a thistle-like flower of the daisy or *Asteraceae* family, and is among the oldest of cultivated plants. Dyes from the plant and seeds have been found in Egyptian tombs, including that of Tutankhamen. Cultivated for its seeds over thousands of years, it is another of the ancient food crops. Used as medicine, dye, food, and oil, safflower is an ancient and versatile plant.

Hybridization and natural mutations have created different varieties of safflower seeds. Naturally high in linoleic acid, hybrids are predominantly high in oleic acid, and produce high-oleic safflower oil. Both high-linoleic and high-oleic versions are commonly available, one high in polyunsaturated linoleic acid and other in monounsaturated oleic acid. The hi-linoleic acid-containing oil can be substituted for linseed oil in making white paint, as it doesn't darken when dry. Most oils for cooking and cosmetics are of the former, high-oleic composition. Both oils are compatible with the skin and are deeply moisturizing, bringing their own fatty acid qualities to skin care.

INCI — *Carthamus tinctorius (Safflower) Seed Oil*

INCI Soap — *Sodium Safflowerate*

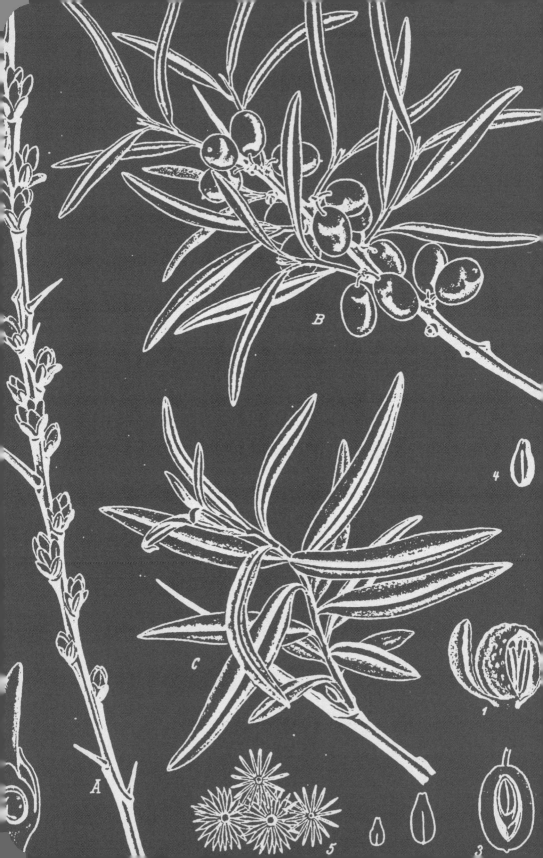

Sea buckthorn oil, *Hippophae Rhamnoides*, with the botanical name *Hippophae*, is from the Greek meaning "shiny horse." Historically fed to Greek horses, the leaves, fruit, and branches made their coats exceptionally shiny and healthy. Pegasus, the mythological flying horse, is said to have favored the leaves of the plant above all other food. Indigenous to Europe and the East, it is a traditional source of food, medicine, and skin care. Sea buckthorn is still used as food and medicine in Russia, Germany, France, Spain, Sweden, Denmark, and Poland. In Mongolia and Tibet, where it figures in traditional healing, it goes by the name Star-Bu or Dhar-Bu.

The pulp of the Sea Buckthorn **berries** are a storehouse of nutrition, rich in vitamins, minerals, and nutrients. The berries are low in oil content, with only 12 to 15% of predominantly monounsaturated fatty acids. Traditional methods of extraction centered on maceration in a fixed oil. Super critical CO_2 extraction methods have made highly concentrated extracts available, consisting of the lipids, vitamins, minerals, and plant waxes. These are called a *total,* and are a concentrated product containing the beneficial properties of the pulp.

Sea buckthorn **seeds** have a different fatty acid composition than the pulp and are high in the omega-3 and omega-6 essential fatty acids. Combining the two extractions makes an exceptionally nourishing oil and skin care supplement.

Traditional uses of sea buckthorn include treatment of the digestive system and in food preparation. For skin conditions, it has the ability to promote regeneration of skin cells and mucous membranes, heal wounds, and ease pain. Its powerful orange color, high in the provitamin A carotenes and carotenoids, is able to protect against damaging UV exposure. Vitamin E tocopherols, vitamin C and flavonoids, vitamins B1, B2, and K, as well as essential fatty acids and phytosterols, make sea buckthorn an exceptionally nourishing ingredient in caring for the skin.

⤶ **Sea Buckthorn**

INCI—*Hippophae Rhamnoides (Sea Buckthorn) Fruit Oil*

INCI—*Hippophae Rhamnoides (Sea Buckthorn) Seed Oil*

INCI—*Hippophae Rhamnoides (Sea Buckthorn) Oil*

Sesame seed oil (*Sesamum indicum*), considered one of humanity's oldest seed crops and cultivated in India for over 5,000 years, is used for cooking and medical purposes. With a very high oil content, the seeds grow under extreme conditions of drought and hardship. Ayurvedic medicine makes extensive use of the oil and the equally ancient Ebers Papyrus of Egypt includes sesame in the list of medicines.

Sesame oil is antibacterial for common skin pathogens, fungi, and athlete's foot. It is naturally anti-inflammatory and a potent antioxidant that can neutralize oxygen radicals in the lower skin layers. Easily absorbed by the skin, sesame oil carries healing properties to the capillaries at the lowest skin layers. As a cell growth regulator, it has been shown to be helpful against cancer cells, and is considered a natural protector against sun damage and UV exposure. The oil has been preliminarily assigned an SPF of 15 but extensive testing has yet to be done. Additionally, some accounts tell of its ability to eradicate lice from the scalp and hair.

Phytosterols found in sesame, *sesamol* and *sesamin,* are natural preservatives that are specific to sesame. They help preserve its linoleic acid content (42%) from oxidation, making it a good choice for herbal oil extractions. Anti-inflammatory and moisturizing, its lignans help modulate the production of sebum, a benefit to acne sufferers. Raw sesame oil is mild-smelling and light-colored. To make toasted sesame oil, common in Asian cooking, the seeds are roasted before pressing. The resulting oil has a strong toasted scent, great for cooking but a bit heavy for skin care. When purchasing sesame oil for body care and extractions, find the unrefined oil, not the toasted version. However, both forms of the oil can be used for low-heat cooking and flavoring.

INCI — *Sesamum indicum (Sesame) Oil*

As a soap oil, sesame is beneficial for the skin and combines well in a formula balanced with saturated and unsaturated oils. Sesame oil infused with herbs can be added to soap to give the bars color and herbal properties.

INCI Soap — *Sodium Sesamate*

Shea butter, known as *Butyrospermum parkii*, has been recently

assigned a new botanical name, *Vitellaria paradoxa*. Also known as African karite butter, it is extracted from the nuts of the shea or karite tree. In the same family as argan and native to Africa, the tree is used by native populations for a wide variety of applications. Native healers have traditionally used shea for muscle aches and strains, arthritis, and skin treatments, while drummers use the butter on their hands to protect them from cracks, dryness, and hard use caused by hours of drumming. Even the drumheads are conditioned with the butter. Used for cooking, general skin care, and sun protection, shea butter is integral to the native way of life.

Shea butter has the highest ratio (up to 17%) of unsaponifiable compounds of all the vegetable fats or oils. These unsaponifiable elements are rich in vitamins, plant sterols, minerals, and other nourishing compounds for the skin and body. The butter softens, protects against drying, and nourishes the skin. Rich in the phenolic compound cinnamic acid and high in tocopherol vitamin E content, the butter is able to protect against the sun's rays and resist oxidation.

Shea butter also has properties that increase local capillary circulation in the skin, helping with oxygenation of tissues. This helps clear the skin by removing metabolic waste products. Saturated fatty acids provide protection, preventing moisture loss, while the oleic and linoleic acids moisturize and maintain the skin's elasticity. Shea butter is particularly protective against the elements and nourishing to the skin where it is applied.

Shea butter can be found in refined and unrefined forms, which are very different in texture, scent, and active properties. The unrefined butter is preferred for therapeutic applications and it tends to remains fresh longer. In time, refined butter develops a sharp unpleasant smell, because many of the protective unsaponifiable elements have been removed. The unrefined version's high content of unsaponifiable compounds makes a superior superfatting agent for soap-making.

INCI — *Butyrospermum Parkii (Shea Butter) Fruit*

INCI Soap — *Sodium Shea Butterate*

Shea oil, *Butyrospermum Parkii,* is produced from the same tree and nuts as the butter. The butter is often listed as stearin, in contrast to the oil, which is listed as olein; each are products from different phases of the extraction process. The seeds are first broken, cold-pressed, and followed by light refinement, then as the butter is being extracted by heat, a liquid oil appears. This liquid olein is separated from the butter stearins to produce oil.

As an oil, shea is high in oleic acid, whereas the butter is high in saturated stearic and palmitic acids. It is a thick, beautiful oil, with the feel of heavy liquid richness. Like other vegetable oils, it pours at room temperature and makes a good massage oil, either mixed with other oils or on its own. With its luxurious rich feel, the oil is excellent for treating skin issues, burns, irritation, and dryness, and in massage. Lighter than the butter, the oil mixes well into recipes.

INCI — *Butyrospermum Parkii Seed Oil*

Shea nilotica, *Vitellaria paradoxa, subsp.* To consumers in the West, *Shea Nilotica* is a new variety of butter from a related species of tree that grows wild in the eastern region of Africa, northern Uganda, and southern Sudan. Known in English as the Nilotica shea tree, nuts are harvested locally and pressed for the butter. Nilotica shea butter, softer than the West African variety, is pale yellow with a high olein content that comes from a glyceride of oleic acid, giving it a softer and creamier texture. High in unsaponifiables, antioxidants, and cinnamic acid, it protects against UV rays. Fairly well absorbed into the skin, the butter will be both protective and nourishing, providing compounds similar to the more common shea. With a lower melting point and less waxy feel, the nilotica shea butter will liquify in warm temperatures and can be easily spread on the skin.

INCI— *Vitellaria Nilotica (Shea) Fruit Butter*

Soybean oil, *Soja hispida,* is very high in unsaturated fatty acids (over 50% linoleic acid) when untreated. Much of the soybean oil produced is hydrogenated because of the oil's polyunsaturated fatty acid makeup, which would cause it to go rancid quickly—nine billion pounds a year is produced in the United States alone. Genetic modification, hydrogenation, and conventional farming practices render it an oil to be avoided for natural skin care, unless it is grown and handled as an organic product.

Before being hydrogenated, soybean oil is high in vitamin E (approximately 30 IU per ounce) and sterolins, which are skin-softening. Grown organically and unrefined, soybeans are high in lecithin and phospholipids. The lecithin is often removed as a valuable by-product and sold separately. Organic certification insures the oil is wholesome enough for natural and organic soap, medicine, and cosmetic-making. Adding vitamin E will stabilize the high linoleic acid content of the oil.

INCI—*Glycine Soja (Soybean) Oil*

INCI Soap—*Sodium Soybeanate*

Shortening, often made from soybean oil, was introduced originally as a fat replacement for lard, as margarine replaced butter. It is familiar in many kitchens and can be used to make soap. The oil undergoes a process of hydrogenation, making an unsaturated oil saturated, or solid, at room temperature. This alters its natural state and in the process destroys beneficial and nutritional properties. In soap, it contributes bulk, saturated fatty acids for easy saponification, mildness, and a stable lather, but is low in nutritional benefits.

INCI—*Sodium Soybeanate*

Natural shortenings with no hydrogenation or trans fats consist of naturally saturated palm oil. Packaged for cooking, they are a return to palm oils' traditional use in Africa as a cooking fat. Use a palm oil SAP for formulating soap recipes.

INCI Soap—*Sodium Palmate*

Sunflower oil, *Helianthus annus*, is pressed from the flowers of several hybridized sunflower varieties. Crop and seed hybridization yields different fatty acid structures, high-oleic, high-linoleic, and mid-oleic, for the food and cosmetics industries. As the name suggests, high- and mid-oleic oils are higher in monounsaturated fatty acids, thus more stable than the high-linoleic. The high-linoleic version, with its unsaturated fatty acids, is used for making paint and other industrial uses. It is suitable for skin care and in food preparation but needs protection from oxidation.

Sunflower oils are inexpensive and useful for cosmetics and soap making.

Their effect on the skin varies by the fatty acid composition of the oil used. Sunflower oil has a fair amount of vitamin E naturally, and that will protect it against rancidity. The high-oleic type oil will tolerate longer storage than the high-linoleic variety. Check the manufacturer's SAP value before formulating soap recipes, as the different hybrids will have different saponification values.

INCI — *Helianthus annus (Sunflower) Seed Oil*

INCI Soap—*Sodium Sunflowerate*

Tamanu see **Caulophyllum Inophyllum**

Tomato seed oil, *Solanum lycopersicum*, is a newer oil on the market that has many of the beneficial properties of the fruit. With an essential fatty acid composition of 50% linoleic acid, antioxidants, vitamins, minerals, carotenes including lycopene, phytosterols, proteins, and lecithin, it is a storehouse of important nutrients. The most nutritious parts of the fruit, tomato skin and seeds, are leftovers from making tomato sauce and juice. Rather than discarding this tomato pomace, it is pressed for its valuable oil and nutrients. Abundant antioxidant compounds, flavonoids, vitamins E and C, essential amino acids, copper, iron, and manganese in this oil provide a high level of nourishment for the skin.

Able to penetrate and support the skin against the usual signs of aging thanks to its high level of plant compounds, the oil is exceptionally nourishing. Its deep orange color indicates a high carotene and lycopene content, able to provide natural UV protection and the ability to repair sun-damaged skin. Nourishing compounds and 25% palmitic acid lend a stability to the oil that helps preserve products while also nourishing and protecting the skin. The oil has a smoky, spicy scent, and delivers a nutrient-dense therapeutic application used in products and for massage.

Turkey red oil, or sulfated castor oil, *Ricinus*

communis, is castor oil that has been treated with the salt of sulfuric acid to make it disperse in water. Turkey red oil was the first *surfactant*, surface-active agent, manufactured in the nineteenth century. (Surfactants are emulsifying and wetting agents.) A common use for turkey red oil is in the making of dispersing bath oils and hair products. In water it is miscible, meaning that it dissolves into a tub of water without separating out.

INCI— *Sulfated Castor Oil*

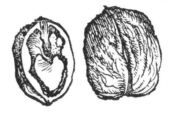

Walnut oil, *Juglans regia,* is a highly unsaturated oil classed as one

of the drying oils. As such, walnut oil needs protection from heat and light to prevent it going rancid. The desire for natural ingredients in art materials has resulted in a line of walnut oil-based paints for artists. This is a plus, as walnut oil does not dry with a yellow cast the way linseed oil does.

Walnut oil is high in poly and superunsaturated fatty acids and plant compounds that are able to nourish the skin and provide anti-aging, regenerative, and moisturizing properties. High in antioxidant ellagic acid, it has anti-bacterial, anti-inflammatory, antiviral, and antiseptic properties, and has shown the ability to suppress tumor growth. Its gallic acid and malic acid are also antioxidants, but are present in lesser amounts. Rich in phytonutrients, walnuts are an excellent source of selenium, phosphorous, magnesium, zinc, iron, and calcium—all food for the skin. Walnut oil is toning and can be used in a variety of skin care preparations. Combined with vitamin E and other more stable oil combinations, it produces skin care that nourishes and supports skin tissues.

INCI—*Juglans Regia (Walnut) Seed Oil*

Walnut oil, low in unsaponifiables and very unsaturated, needs to be balanced with saturated oils to help it saponify. Adding walnut oil to soap is said to increase the hardness factor of the final bars by measurable amounts.

INCI Soap—*Sodium Walnutate*

Watermelon seed oil, *Citrullus vulgaris,* known as *ootanga oil, tsamma* (a local name), or *kalahari oil,* may be a new oil in the West but has a long tradition in Africa as an indigenous traditional oil. The first recorded harvest is 5,000 years old and is represented in Egyptian heiroglyphs. The oil originates in the Kalahari desert from native and moisture-rich melons. The local women grow the fruit, carefully collecting the seeds and taking them to a mill for pressing to extract the oil. Used for cooking, dressings, skin, and hair care, the oil is a central part of native life.

High in linoleic acid (as much as 65%), watermelon seed oil is exceptionally light and highly nutritious. It absorbs well and is used for troubled skin, helping to dissolve excessive sebum in the pores and repairing damage to the cells. Anti-inflammatory, it helps relieve the pain associated with acne eruptions and conditions. Its very lightness is helpful for conditioning oily skin and helps to minimize pore size.

Watermelon oil is very high in the B vitamins, especially niacin, along with the minerals magnesium and zinc. It nourishes and repairs without clogging pores. The light oil can be used on babies and for mature skin care repair and rejuvenation. A highly stable oil with a long shelf life, it is added to recipes to help preserve products. Its light feel makes a good oil for combining with heavier oils, and its light texture makes it a recommended natural replacement for mineral oil.

INCI— *Citrullus vulgaris (Watermelon) Seed Oil*

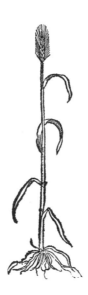

Wheat germ oil, *Triticum vulgare*, is another oil high in unsaponifiable fractions and essential fatty acids, with 55% linoleic acid. Rich in sterols and high in antioxidant activity due to its natural vitamin E content, the oil is able to protect the lipids of the skin from free radical damage. With a squalene content at close to 1%, wheat germ oil helps repair and support weather and sun-damaged skin. Phytosterols, beta-sitosterols, and campesterol are anti-inflammatory and protect the barrier function, while ferulic acid, tocopherols, and carotenoids protect against sun and weather damage.

Topical applications of wheat germ oil improve circulation close to the skin's surface and strengthen the connective tissue, helping maintain the skin's elasticity. Its positive effect on cellular formation facilitates regeneration and repair by healing cuts and abrasions, and providing moisturizing and conditioning properties.

INCI— *Triticum vulgare (Wheat) Germ Oil*

INCI Soap— *Sodium Wheatgermate*

Yangu, Cape Chestnut, *Calodendrum capense,* a native
of South Africa, is not related to the chestnut, but appeared that way to early explorers who gave the plant its name. Yangu is said to be a beautiful African forest tree. "Oil of the Massai," produced by the Maasai tribe and distributed by a company in the US, is helping to preserve the tribe's habitat and way of life. A popular oil in Africa for skin care, yangu has natural sun-screening and skin protective properties. With oleic acid at 45%, the oil is conditioning and protective of the outer skin layers. Yangu is rich in antioxidants and essential fatty acids, with linoleic acid at 30% giving it qualities that protect the lipid barrier and hold moisture in the skin.

INCI— *Calodendrum Capense (Yangu) Oil*

Natural Waxes Used in Skin Care

Plants produce waxes for protection. Whether it's a harsh climate, dryness, intense wetness, heat, cold, even invasion by insects or small animals, waxes help to seal plant tissues from the surrounding, sometimes hostile, environment. Waxes can be produced in many parts of the plant, including the leaves, stem, trunk, nuts, and kernels. They are lipids, fatty acids possessing protective and nutitional properties for the plant. Animals also produce waxes that we use in foods and skin care. Naturally formed waxes, whether from plants or animals, are more compatible with our physiologic functions than synthetic versions.

ANIMAL WAXES

Beeswax is obtained from the honeycomb of the honeybee, *Apis mellifera*. Beeswax has been used for thousands of years as medicine and especially in the fine arts. Before the nineteenth century, any references to a wax was exclusively a reference to beeswax. To obtain beeswax, honeycombs of the beehive are removed and the honey extracted. Then the wax comb is melted in boiling water, filtered, and made into cakes or cast into forms.

Beeswax comes in both white and yellow forms, which are interchangeable in cosmetics. The type of flower the hive visited determines the color of the wax. Yellow beeswax can also be bleached with oxidizing agents to form a white wax for the cosmetic industry, which often prefers a wax without color or scent. The wax is used as a thickener and in the emulsion process for making creams. Beeswax added to oils creates salves, solid lipid combinations that can be aromatic perfumes or herbal medicines. By using different proportions of wax to oil, salves can be hard and stand alone, or soft and contained in a jar. The melting point of beeswax is 143.6°–149°.

INCI — *Cera Alba*

Lanolin, or **wool wax**, is often used in skin care products and is a fatty secretion from the wool of sheep. This wool wax is completely different from the body fat of the sheep, having a soft texture. Secreted from special sebaceous glands in the animal's skin, it forms a protective coating on the wool fibers. The name lanolin comes from the latin *lana* for wool, and *oleum*, oil, and consists of long-chain waxy sterol esters. It lacks the glycerol esters of the triglycerides, so is not a true oil or fat. Interestingly, however, lanolin has similar properties to the stratum corneum lipids that govern and regulate the water content of the skin.

The crude wax is extracted from the fleece by various washing processes, then refined for use. Lanolin is often seen in two forms: hydrous, meaning that it has water in it, and anhydrous, which is pure wool wax without water present. Lanolin has been used in skin care products and for industrial uses as a lubricant and for waterproofing for hundreds of years.

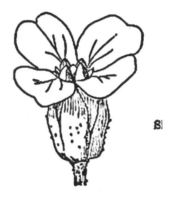

BOTANICAL WAXES

Candelilla Wax, *Euphorbiea Cerifera,* is a vegetable wax from a reed-type plant growing in southern Texas and northern Mexico. The mature uprooted plant is boiled in acidified water, the wax rising to the top. It is then skimmed off the surface and hardened into forms. The wax is light tan to yellow, and comes in lump and pellet forms. Its melting point is 155°–162°, and it has commercial uses in cosmetics, foods, and pharmaceuticals. The FDA has designated candelilla wax as GRAS—Generally Recognized As Safe—for use in foods.

INCI— *Euphorbiea Cerifera (Candelilla) Wax*

Carnauba Wax, *Copernica cerifera,* is a natural exudate from the fronds of the Brazilian palm tree. The plant conserves moisture within the leaves and trunk, using the wax as protection. *Arbol del Vida,* or "Tree of Life" in its native Brazil, provides many products and serves many traditional uses for the native population. There are carnauba palms in several counties, but because of weather conditions, only one area in the semi-arid northeast section of Brazil grows the trees that produce 80% of the carnauba wax on the market.

The fronds are cut and dried before the wax is mechanically removed. Melting and filtering removes impurities in the raw product. The wax is naturally various shades of yellow and its melting point is 181.4° and higher, making it a very hard wax. The high melting point creates a wax that can be polished and buffed to a high shine, which is why it is found in floor and furniture polishes. The commercial uses of carnauba wax include a polishing agent for candies, pills, and leather, in casting techniques, and in cosmetics. The FDA has classified it as GRAS, Generally Recognized As Safe, for use in foods.

INCI — *Copernica cerifera (Carnauba) Wax*

Castor wax, *Ricinus communis,* a hydrogenated wax from castor oil, is a hard, brittle wax used for making cosmetic stick products such as lipsticks, eye pencils, and others. Castor oil is made by bubbling hydrogen through the oil with a nickel catalyst that hardens the oil, making it solid. Castor wax has a melting point of 70°C or 158°F.

INCI — *Ricinus communis (Castor) Wax*

Japan wax, *Rhus verniciflua* and other *Rhus* species, is a wax derived from the berries of a small tree native to the Japanese islands. Called *Moku-ro* in Japan, this dark green wax is extracted from the crushed berries, which are boiled and pressed. The raw wax, *Ki-ro*, is used for making candles, styling traditional wigs, and for industrial uses. The refined wax, *Moku Row*, is extracted of impurities and refined by sunlight and water into a pure white wax. This refined wax is used in lipsticks, medicines, crayons, industrial goods, and ointments. Chemically, Japan wax is not a true wax, being composed of glycerides and free palmitic acids. It is more like a stiff oil, perhaps a counterpart to jojoba, which is a liquid wax.

Jojoba wax (ho-ho-ba), *Simmondsia chinensis*, is similar to jojoba butter, but the melting point is raised further by hydrogenation, producing a hard, waxy substance. Jojoba wax is used primarily in the production of cosmetics, candles, and other specialty items. The melting point varies, determined by the degree of processing, from hard waxes to various levels of softness of butters.

INCI — *Simmondsia chinensis (Jojoba) Wax*

Ouricury wax, *Syagros coronata*, from the brazilian feather palm, is similar to carnauba wax but more difficult to harvest, as the wax must be stripped off the plant by hand rather than flaking off naturally as the carnauba wax does. It can be used as a replacement for carnauba, but is darker in color when applied.

INCI — *Syagros coronata (Ouricury) Wax*

Rice bran wax, *Oryza sativa,* is extracted from crude rice bran oil. The oil is de-gummed, and the fatty acid content reduced by solvent extraction, leaving a wax behind. Rice bran wax may be used in some food applications but it does not carry the GRAS designation.

INCI — *Oryza sativa (Rice Bran) Wax*

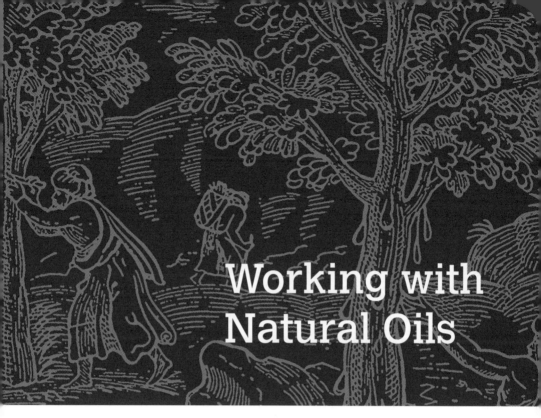

Working with Natural Oils

Now that we've learned all about the different types of oil and vegetable butters, it's time to apply what we've learned. Time to get our hands dirty—or oily in our case—roll up the sleeves, grab an apron, and begin. There are almost endless ways of working with the oils, including creating soaps, massage oils, salves, ointments, balms, creams, lotions, and perfumes. Because the subject is so large, enough to spawn another book, we'll focus on working only with the oils and leave the soaps and composite products like creams alone for now.

Care and Handling of Oils

Natural oils possess a life-like quality, especially when fresh. Sourced from living seeds and kernels, some are durable and stable, while others are more delicate, reacting with the air and environment. Handling oils properly insures that they remain wholesome and that their properties are preserved while you use them. Good handling practices apply to all oils: avoid heat, light, and air as much as you can, and use the oils in a timely manner.

Storage is an especially important part of good handling. We've learned that heat and light will transform polyunsaturated oils into new states, oxidizing them and turning them rancid. All oils should be stored at moderate temperatures, no higher than 70 degrees in a dark cupboard or room, with very polyunsaturated oils best stored under refrigeration to prolong their useful life. The best type of storage system will depend on the oil being stored and the length of time kept before use.

> ❀ Saturated solid oils (coconut, shea, and the tropical butters) are the most hardy and stable, able to handle warmer conditions and light for a period of time. Refrigeration is not usually necessary to store these types of oil.

> ❀ The predominately monounsaturated oils (olive, sesame, avocado, and others) hold up well in normal living temperatures (around 70 degrees) when stored in dark bottles for several months up to a year.

> ❀ The poly (grape-seed, evening primrose, walnut) and super polyunsaturated oils (flax, chia, hemp, and others) need to be kept in a dark area, in closed containers, and under refrigeration if possible.

Purchase oils as you need them. Unlike most essential oils, which can last many years, fixed oils shouldn't be hoarded. They will, however, store well for about six months, and with cold storage most will last much longer. If you purchase gallon and five-gallon quantities, smaller amounts can be drawn off for day-to-day use while the larger volume is kept cool and dark.

There are many excellent suppliers of oils, both organic and conventional, at a wide variety of prices. Choosing a supplier will depend on the quality and price of the oil desired and the shipping distance. Oils are heavy, and shipping costs are based on weight. A slightly higher-priced oil closer to home beats a great price from across the country. That is, as long as the quality is comparable.

Food-grade oils are distributed by suppliers certified to handle food products. The requirements for facilities and handling are more stringent, and more closely monitored. Distributors of cosmetic-grade oils haven't undergone the further certification to become food approved. Both sources of oil can be used in cosmetics and for external applications.

Using Oils on the Skin

Applying oils and vegetable butters to the body has untold benefits for the skin. Liquid or solid, all oils protect the skin and body from weather and dryness. Natural properties of warmth and energy provide protection for the skin tissues. In cold climates or during cold winter months, oils help to retain natural body warmth by keeping moisture locked inside the skin and body. Using and combining oils to protect, warm, or nourish the skin is where the magic begins.

Olive oil from the kitchen cabinet makes a great suntan oil. Coconut oil is used for all manner of personal care from toothpaste and deodorant to massage and face care. The liquid oils can be used on their own for massage treatments, for moisturizing, skin protection, or to condition the skin after the bath. The solid oils and butters can be rubbed into the skin on their own for occlusive protection and for moisturizing. Salves, ointments, body butters, scrubs, balms—the list only ends when your imagination does. The following combinations and recipes will get you started. But don't stop with our ideas—get to know the oils and make your own combinations.

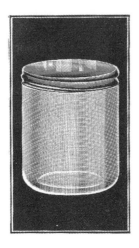

Facial Care with Natural Oils

Our faces are our window to the world. We face the day, put our face forward, and about-face when necessary! Some of us even put our faces on in the morning. Facial care that enhances our native beauty need be no more exotic than gently caring for the skin with food-grade nutrients. Natural ingredients that spring from the plants and earth speak to our skin and body in a language it can understand. Synthetic chemicals are just so much junk food and a language so foreign as to not be recognizable to our tissues. They may appear to help in the short term, but over the long term the skin grays and looses vitality. Natural plant-based oils, our favorite subject, are an excellent source of great skin care.

CLEANSING WITH OILS

Soap and running water are a recent phenomena in the evolution of human culture, improving hygiene and our standard of living. The availability of hot showers and soap led to the abandonment of the ancient practice of oil cleansing. Now we squeaky-clean our skin, then turn around and moisturize it to replace its natural oil balance.

Our skin is made up of and produces a variety of lipids; the outermost layer is well over 60% fatty acid lipids. Oil protects the cell walls, fights bacteria, heals wounds, alleviates irritation, and prevents moisture from evaporating from the skin layers. By washing all the natural oils off the skin, it must spring into action to replace what was lost. Oil cleansing is a way of both cleaning the skin and keeping it moisturized and supple. With oil cleansing, older, hardened oils in the skin are dissolved and the skin refreshed with new oils. The skin does not have to over-work to make up what was lost by soap and water washing.

Our ancestors can teach us a few beneficial ancient practices. The Greeks, Romans, and Egyptians used oil to cleanse the skin. Oil was applied generously and massaged into the body, the excess scraped away with a blunt tool along with dirt and dead skin cells. Afterward, fresh oil was applied to keep the skin protected against weather and harsh climates. Olive was the oil overwhelmingly used around the Mediterranean, while people in tropical Africa or South America use native oils such as shea and palm.

The use of oils to clean the skin is being rediscovered. The first step to begin using this method of cleansing is to find an oil—used singly or in combination—suited to your own skin type.

HOW TO OIL CLEANSE

There are two possible methods. For the first method, take a good dollop of oil in the palm of the hand and rub the hands together. Apply oil to dry skin on the face and neck, and thoroughly massage into the skin. The oil will lift makeup, along with dirt and dead skin cells. When the face is fully covered with oil, place a hot (but not so hot it burns) washcloth, wrung out, over the skin. This step allows the pores of the skin to open and release oils and debris. After a minute or two wipe or rinse the excess oil from the face. Pat the skin dry, and it will feel quite dry in a few minutes, even after having used all that oil. Then apply a nourishing facial oil to maintain moisture in the tissues.

The second method involves using a little hydrosol or pure water with the oil in the palm of the hand. Rub them together vigorously to create a kind of impromptu emulsion, apply to the face, and proceed as above.

OIL CLEANSING BY FATTY ACID TYPE

Any of the wide range of fatty acid types and their oils can be used for oil cleansing. The feel and results will differ depending on your skin type, the climate you live in, and the time of year.

Unless it is extremely dry, our skin will produce more oils in the warmer months and climates than in winter's very cold and dry temperatures. Native peoples of the polar regions use saturated animal fats for protection against cold chapping air. People of tropical regions where the sun is intense use native saturated butters as protection against excessive rays of the sun. In the temperate regions, lighter and less saturated oils are preferred. They "wash" off more easily and leave the skin ready for a cream or facial oil and make-up, if worn.

The more unsaturated an oil's fatty acids, the greater the ability of the skin to absorb the oil into the tissues. Oils high in both essential fatty acids are absorbed the most readily. Oils high in omega-6 linoleic acid follow just behind the more unsaturated oils.

Monounsaturated oils are a bit heavier than the more unsaturated omega-6 and 3 oils and will stay on the surface of the skin longer. They are more able to really loosen makeup, dirt, and oil produced by the skin. The very-long-chain fatty acid type oils, such as meadowfoam and moringa oils, twenty carbon atoms long and above, are much heavier-feeling, and less able to penetrate quickly, but serve the skin as emollients and as protective agents. They may be wiped off to achieve a light moisturized feel when done.

Commercial blends are available as well, but you can easily make your own. See the suggestions below, or consult the fatty acid tables at the back of the book to find a combination that suits your skin type, season, and weather exposure.

SUGGESTIONS FOR OILS TO CLEANSE THE SKIN

Dry Skin

❀ High monounsaturated oils such as olive, avocado, macadamia, almond, sesame, and camellia. Jojoba oil is an excellent "oil" for all skin types, although it is technically a wax.

❀ For very dry skin, use oils high in oleic and some saturated fatty acids, such as palmitic acid. Try papaya seed oil, shea oil, or macadamia.

Normal Skin

❀ Oils with balanced oleic and linoleic acid levels work well here, such as cranberry seed, apricot kernel, argan, and baobab. Jojoba oil also works well. Coconut oil, too, with its medium chain fatty acids is light, absorbs somewhat, and can be washed away.

Oily Skin

❀ The following oils high in omega-3 and 6 fatty acids help to calm, replenish, and normalize. Use them singly or in combination: camelina, chia seed, sacha inchi, kiwi seed, blackberry, kukui, raspberry, flax, and perilla. Jojoba's lack of triglycerides is especially helpful for skin that over-produces oil. Castor oil is also great for normal and oily skin: it penetrates easily, washes off and helps dry the skin of excess oil. Oils high in tannins are astringent and able to calm over-active oil glands; camellia and hazelnut are two examples.

Blemished Skin

❀ Oils high in omega-6 linoleic acid are best for blemished and challenged skin, soaking into the skin layers and replenishing missing fatty acids. Grapeseed oil is high in omega-6 fatty acids and will replenish the cells of the skin with this often-missing element. Other good options include watermelon, cucumber, evening primrose, and passion fruit seed oils.

ESSENTIAL OILS AND OIL CLEANSING

Oil cleansing can incorporate scents with essential oils or not. Oil straight from the bottle works well, but essential oils have therapeutic qualities that can help heal skin conditions or enliven a dull complexion.

⊛ A mild eucalyptus such as radiata, helichrysum, or chamomile can help control inflamed tissues.

⊛ Lavender can soothe the nervous system while toning and calming skin.

⊛ The very elegant and expensive rose otto or neroli essential oils are made for beautiful skin care.

Consult one of the many great books on essential oils for more suggestions on essential oils for facial care (see the bibliography and more information below).

REMOVING EYE MAKE-UP

Use a bit of oil like grape-seed, evening primrose, or coconut on a cotton ball or tissue to wipe away mascara, shadow, and liner. Take care to not get the oil in the eye, as it will leave a light film and cloud the eye for a few minutes. Some oils will irritate slightly if eye contact is made, so use just the lightest amount to gently dissolve and wipe away makeup from lids and lashes.

Note, it is best to remove contact lenses when using oil to remove eye make up. The oil may get on the lenses and impair your vision. Be sure any oil is gone from the eye before putting your lenses in.

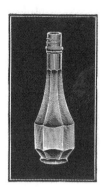

FACIAL OILS OR OIL SERUMS

With the wide variety of oils available, beautiful and nourishing combinations can be created to feed the skin a diet high in antioxidants, vitamins, minerals, and high-quality lipids. First, determine what you want to supply to the skin: Vitamin C or vitamin E? Antioxidants for protection from the sun, perhaps? Anti-aging compounds to slow the effects of environment and time? The following are a few recipe ideas to begin the discovery process. If not all the oils are available, substitute or leave them out of the mix. Keep track of your proportions and take notes so that you can duplicate or modify the combinations you make.

Facial oils and oil serums are designed to absorb into the skin quickly. The more unsaturated an oil, the more quickly it can be absorbed by the skin. Fatty acid chain length, too, makes a difference in absorption, with shorter chains more easily received by the tissues than longer ones. Base your facial oil on the essential fatty acids, omega-3 and 6, for quick penetration of the skin. Add smaller amounts of nutrient-dense omega-9 fatty acid oils for their ability to provide beneficial compounds that feed and support skin cells. The recipe ideas include essential oil suggestions; a place to start but not the end. Use only a few drops for scent and toning—a little goes a long way.

MAKING AND USING OIL SERUMS

General tips:

✾ Use high quality oils, organic if possible for their greater nutrient content.

✾ Make up just enough to last a month or two. Remember, many oils can go rancid easily.

✾ Use daily for best results.

✾ Keep combinations cool and dark. Brown or blue bottles work well.

Application:

✾ Applying the oils to damp clean skin is the best method, as the oils will absorb easily and quickly. Oil will help lock in the moisture that remains from cleansing.

Seasonality:

Cold weather

✾ Cold winter temperatures are often accompanied by extremely dry air. The skin must struggle to maintain moisture in the cells. Applying facial oils will help keep moisture in by providing a lipid barrier between outside environment and the skin tissues. Be sure and drink plenty of water to supply moisture on the inside as well.

Summer

✾ Hot and humid climates or seasons often have an opposite effect, and the skin over-produces sebum and moisture in the form of sweat. Additional oils aren't necessarily needed on days like these, however, oils are helpful for providing protection from the sun, introducing antioxidant compounds or tightening the skin with the dry-feeling oils.

✳ Hot and dry environmental conditions call for oils that protect and keep moisture in the skin. Here, oils that are grown under similar weather—like jojoba or argan—help protect cells from extremely dry conditions.

SCENTING

Scenting your serum or facial oil is part of delicious skin care. Please use good-quality essential oils that have therapeutic value for the skin and body. The following recipes include suggestions, or research your own in the many publications on essential oils available (my favorites are listed in the bibliography). To get you started, the following essential oils are especially beneficial for the skin and face: rose, lavender, geranium, neroli, chamomile, rosemary verbenone, carrot seed, myrrh, ylang ylang, and lemon verbena. One caution: the citrus oils are lovely scents, but most can have photosensitizing effects on the skin in the presence of strong sunlight. Use the citrus oils in wash-off products for their enlivening properties.

CONTAINERS

Liquid oil serums are often packaged in small bottles of one ounce or less. A dropper top or dispenser cap helps deliver just a small amount of oil to the skin, where it can be massaged in easily. Solid oils (also known as butters) are better packaged in open-mouth jars or tins. However, some saturated combinations liquefy in the heat and can be used in bottles or squeeze containers. Experiment with your combination.

COMBINING YOUR MIXTURES

The following recipe suggestions are listed by parts. Determine the volume you want to create, and divide by the number of ingredients you plan to use of equal measure. Make it easy and work in whole or half parts.

⊛ For personal use, a part could be ½ ounce (one tablespoon), or 1 ounce (two tablespoons).

⊛ For bulk production, use parts up to 4 or more ounces.

Note: it is better to make fresh batches than have a large amount go bad.

Mixing the liquid oils together can be done in a small measuring cup or beaker, and the result poured through a funnel and into a bottle. Always label your productions. Speaking from experience, a week or month from now that little bottle will be a mystery.

Solid oil combinations using the butters are gently melted together and poured into open mouth jars for easy dispensing.

PRESERVING YOUR SERUMS

Some oils are so stable naturally that they can help preserve a formula from oxidation. Meadowfoam, marula, moringa, and baobab are oils with strong preserving properties and can be added to combinations to help protect your formula. Vitamin E also preserves oils from oxidation. Extracted from oils high in the vitamin, vitamin E comes in different levels of concentration. The amount to use in a formula is determined by the strength of the extract. A note of caution: some people are sensitive to the vitamin in concentration.

USING YOUR SERUMS

The serums can be used singly or more than one at a time. Or you can identify the conditions you want to address, and mix a custom blend for that issue.

DOCUMENTATION

Keep notes. You'll be able to repeat your successes, or improve on combinations with good documentation. And label your jars and bottles.

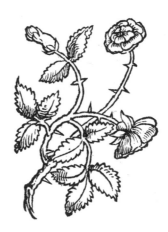

Recipes:

Here are a few suggested combinations to begin with.

Facial Oil for Oily Skin:

Description

Even oily skin needs nourishment and good-quality oils. Astringent oils high in tannins lightly and gently provide a protective layer and calm over-active sebaceous glands.

Examples of dry astringent oils:

Camellia, grape-seed, hazelnut, rice bran, rosehip seed, borage, cranberry seed, jojoba oils, and mango butter. Tamanu added to the mix will help contain blemishes, and prevent scarring. Watermelon seed oil is extremely light and helps clear pores of old fats and debris.

Directions:

Mix several of these oils together and add essential oils that help calm oily skin (see below).

Scents:

Spike lavender, lavender, rosemary verbenone, helichrysum, ylang ylang, or a mild eucalyptus like radiata. Use 6 to 10 drops per ounce.

Use:

Apply a light film to damp clean skin and allow to absorb.

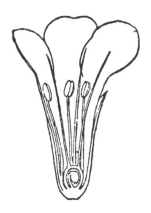

Vitamin C Oil Serum:

Description

Vitamin C is necessary for collagen production and healthy skin. It supports the skin's innate immune function and protects against signs of aging. Oils with exceptional amounts of vitamin C usually come from fruit that is high in the vitamin.

Examples of oils high in vitamin C:

Kiwi, blackberry, rosehip seed, passion fruit, sea buckthorn, blueberry, and black currant.

Directions:

Use equal parts of three or four oils high in the vitamin. Preserve your serum from oxygen by mixing one half part meadowfoam oil or ½ teaspoon per ounce of vitamin E to protect the fatty acids. Put serum in a small dropper bottle or pump and label.

Scents:

Essential oils don't contain vitamin C, so use any pleasing or therapeutic essential oil in your combination. Add a few drops of essential oil, six to 10 drops per ounce (two tablespoons). Neroli is a wonderful complement to the mix.

Anti-Aging Oil Serum:

Description

This serum will protect the skin on multiple levels and help strengthen collagen in the tissues. It features oils high in unsaponifiables and antioxidants.

Examples for base oil:

Equal parts of two or more of avocado, argan, marula, macadamia nut, jojoba, moringa, or pomegranate seed oils.

Extra antioxidant oils:

Add a small amount of buriti, rosehip seed, or sea buckthorn oil. Tamanu oil is a concentrated oil that has many benefits for nourishing tissues and keeping skin happy.

Directions:

To one ounce of the base oils, either in combination or singly, add ½ teaspoon or less of the highly colored antioxidant oils. The highly colored oils will make the skin orange if too much is used. This serum, being high in antioxidants, will resist oxidation, but you can also add vitamin E, about a teaspoon for up to 3 ounces to further protect the oils.

Scent:

Cistus and green myrtle are two essential oils I have used in similar products for mature complexions. Rosemary verbenone, helichrysum, neroli, rose, and geranium are other essential oils beneficial to older complexions as well.

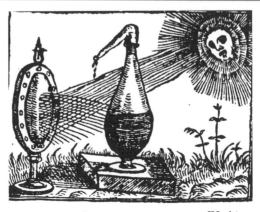

Sun-Protective Oil Serum:

Description

The protection from UV damage is found in the antioxidant compounds that color oils. These compounds mitigate the damaging effects of the sun's rays by protecting against oxidative damage in the skin tissues. Tropical oils and butters are also high in compounds that protect skin from sun damage.

Note of caution:

Sun exposure is important for our health in a number of ways and necessary to make vitamin D in the skin. However, it is also important to protect the skin from burning; long sleeves, shade, hats protect us once our sun exposure reaches its daily optimum. The tropical oils contain sun protection for longer periods of exposure but use common sense and avoid sunburns.

Examples of highly protective oils:

Buriti, carrot seed and root, sea buckthorn, rosehip seed, tomato seed, and oat seed oils. The color indicates the presence of abundant plant-derived antioxidant compounds that mitigate the potential oxidative damage caused by the sun's rays. Examples of tropical sun protective oils are coconut, shea butter, mango butter, babassu, cocoa butter and tamanu.

Directions:

Combine the oils above with base oils like argan, kukui, sesame, jojoba, and meadowfoam or butters such as shea butter, cocoa butter, babassu, or coconut to a desired consistency and color. The highly colored antioxidant oils are diluted in base oils in ratios of 1 part color oil to 6 parts of a base oil, or the equivalent of 1 teaspoon of color oil to ounce of a base. The solid oils need to be melted and thoroughly combined with the liquid oils and scents and allowed to cool and set. Raspberry seed oil is another potential addition; it is currently being studied as especially protective against sun damage.

Scent:

Avoid citrus essential oils for sun exposure to protect the skin from photosensitivity. Lavender, geranium, carrot seed, and lemon verbena oils are some potential additions

Note on use:

Use lavishly when you are going to be in the sun, reapplying often if swimming or perspiring heavily.

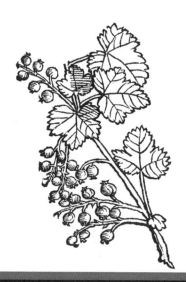

Soothing Oil Serum:

Description

Used on irritated or inflamed skin, this oil has the ability to calm and relieve itching and redness. The avena compounds in oat oil soothe irritation, as does the calming compounds in passion fruit seed oil. The very-long-chain fatty acids of broccoli seed or meadowfoam seed oils will protect skin, and the GLA content of currant or borage seed oils will help reduce redness and irritation.

Caution::

If you are highly sensitive to gluten or have celiac disease, omit the oat oil and add larger quantities of GLA oils (evening primrose, borage, or black currant).

Directions:

Combine equal parts of oat, passion fruit seed, and black currant or borage seed oils. One half part of meadowfoam or broccoli seed oil will help protect the skin from external irritants. For whole body application, the above combination can be diluted with a mild oil like almond, sesame or olive, by half or three quarters.

Scent:

Roman chamomile, lavender, and helichrysum essential oils will help repair and calm the skin.

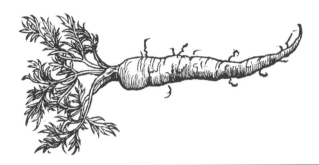

Brightening Facial Oil Serum:

Description

Sometimes the skin becomes dull and pale at the end of a long winter, after too much work or stress, or in the process of switching to a greener, healthier lifestyle. Oils that revitalize the skin can help brighten the complexion

Examples of oils to use to brighten:

Rosehip seed oil, camellia, tomato, sea buckthorn, or cucumber oils.

Oils helpful on skin spots::

Avocado, papaya, rice bran, castor oils.

Directions:

Combine several brightening oils, above, and several of the oils helpful for skin spots, diluting the highly colored oils with those of lighter coloration, usually a 1:6 ratio.

Scents:

Rosemary verbenone, lemon verbena, carrot seed, geranium, and rose are examples of essential oils to revitalize the skin and refresh the complexion.

A cautionary comment: The reason you are making your own combinations is to avoid the many chemicals in personal care products. Using products with synthetic compounds on the skin will devitalize and grey the complexion and can impair your general health. Read the ingredients on any purchased product and avoid if the balance is on non-natural compounds. Most ingredient lists are listed in descending order of volume. That smidgen of herb or natural oil at the bottom of the list is not going to improve the health of the skin.

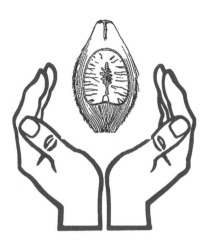

Oils for Massage

Oils used for massage need the right amount of slip so that the hands glide along the skin for the duration of the treatment. But the oil also needs some tack and resistance, so the skin and underlying tissues can be worked. This calls for some oils over others. The following suggestions are general guidelines for useful combinations.

OILS FOR MASSAGE BY FATTY ACID TYPE

See the fatty acid table at the back of the book for suggestions about which oils are strong in the different fatty acids. Here's what the different fatty acids can do:

⊛ Omega-9 oleic acid oils give a good slip on the skin, allowing for some tack as well. Being monounsaturated, these oils do not absorb too quickly into the skin layers.

⊛ Omega-6 linoleic acid-dominant oils tend to absorb into the skin quickly, and need to be reapplied too frequently to be used on their own.

- Omega-3 alpha-Linolenic acid can be mixed with omega-9 oils for skin conditioning, as it absorbs quickly into the skin tissues.

- Saturated oils, such as coconut (fractionated and virgin), are good massage oils. Heavier saturated oils such as shea, cocoa, and mango need to be combined with lighter oils for a good massage treatment.

Some favorite and common massage oils and combinations:

- COCONUT OIL, with its mid-chain fatty acids that melt on contact with the skin, is a good massage oil. It absorbs into the skin but doesn't do so too quickly. Fractionated coconut oil is a liquid version of coconut oil that does not solidify in cold weather and is often used in massage.

- JOJOBA OIL is very compatible with the skin's sebum and another good oil for use in massage.

- OLIVE OIL has been used for massage since Athena gifted it to the ancient Greeks. This one is time-tested, but can have a strong scent reminiscent of salad and food preparation. Choose a refined variety without scent.

- AVOCADO AND ALMOND OILS are similar to olive in fatty acid makeup. High in omega-9 oleic acid, the slip and tack are good and endure.

- MACADAMIA NUT OIL has a strong nutty scent and is high in omega-9 fatty acids. Try a small amount before purchasing in large quantities or dilute with less strongly scented oil.

- SHEA OLEIN is a rich omega-9 oil with saturated fatty acid fractions that give it a rich and luxurious feel. It is a good basic massage choice and can be mixed with other lighter oils to extend their range.

Oils containing tannins, such as camellia, hazelnut, and grape-seed, are better suited for skin care than for massage. They have a dry feeling on the skin that helps repair and tone, but also lacks slip and glide.

Tailoring the oil combination to the person being massaged can improve the massage experience considerably. Use passion fruit seed oil for high-strung or stressed-out individuals or rosehip seed oil on scar tissue. Some oils are particularly beneficial for muscle aches and swellings, such as shea butter in combination with lighter oils like andiroba, papaya, nigella, or passion fruit.

Experimentation with different oils is the best educator. Purchase small amounts, four to eight ounces, and mix and match the textures, the slip, and tack. You will hit on a combination that you, your family, friends and customers will rave about.

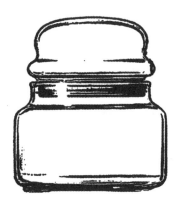

Simple Body Scrubs

Simple and elegant, sugar or salt scrubs on the body do a great job of removing old skin cells, rejuvenating and stimulating the skin for a healthy glow. Add some essential oils or natural color elements and you create a beautiful spa experience at home.

Lemon Salt Scrub

Description

This is a stimulating salt scrub that will exfoliate the skin and improve circulation. Salt crystals gently lift dead skin cells, while lemon essential oil is cleansing and purifying for the skin as well as emotionally uplifting and stress-reducing.

Ingredients:

Fine-textured sea salt or sugar	1 lb.
Sunflower or almond oil	2 to 3 oz. oil
Lemon essential oil	2 tsp (about 200 drops)
Litsea cubeba essential oil	35 drops
Cardamom essential oil	10 drops

Directions:

In a large bowl, put several cups of sea salt or sugar. For every five parts salt or sugar, mix in one part oil sunflower or almond oil. Add your essential oil and mix thoroughly together. Scrubs can be dry, using very little oil, or wet with lots of oil to rub on the skin.

Containers:

If using salt, put in jars with plastic lids. The salt will corrode metal lids and over time, turn the top of your scrub and jar black!

Variations include adding more oil for a wetter, oilier scrub, or less oil for a very dry scrub. Add liquid lecithin, about a teaspoon, and melt into the oil to help the scrub rinse off the skin more easily. Vary the essential oils, add ground seaweed for its minerals and iodine content, or add color clays to draw and cleanse the skin and color the product

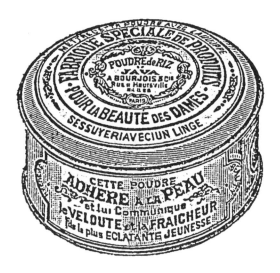

Whipped Salves & Body Butters

These are delightful combinations of saturated and unsaturated oils melted together, cooled and set, then whipped with a kitchen mixer, immersion mixer with whisk attachment, or a hand whisk and very, very strong arm.

Whipped oil combinations can be a bit tricky and will depend in part on the room temperature and season. In summer, when temperatures are high, recipes need to be made with a higher percentage of hard saturated oils like cocoa butter. Cold winter temperatures will work with a softer, less saturated mix. The soft, medium, or hard consistency depends on the temperature of the environment and the proportions of saturated to unsaturated oil. On warm or hot summer days, the whipped mixture can remain quite soft, but harden up as temperatures cool. Too hot, and the oils melt back together and need to be re-whipped.

Recipes in this section are proportional, so they can be increased or decreased as needed. Want just a small amount to try out? Use one ounce for each "part" to get the feel. Making a large tub for gifts? The "parts" can be as much as a pound. Just scale up the vessels used and whip the added volume.

If you find that the combination creates a texture that's too hard, scoop it back into the mixing bowl and add measured liquid oil until it is a better texture. Always measure, so that the recipe can be duplicated if a success or modified if not. Essential oils can be added at any point.

Here are some proportions and their results:

⊛ EQUAL PARTS OF SHEA BUTTER, COCONUT OIL, AND SESAME OIL: makes a very soft mix that remains soft, almost liquid, in cool weather.

⊛ EQUAL PARTS SHEA BUTTER, COCOA BUTTER, AND SESAME OIL: trading the coconut oil in our first example for cocoa butter makes the mix very hard. The level of saturation in the cocoa butter is very high in long-chained saturated fatty acids that are very hard at room temperature. As a variation on this, trade out the cocoa butter for kokum; the mix is very, very hard as well.

⊛ EQUAL PARTS OF BABASSU, COCONUT, AND SESAME: soft in warm weather, sets up in cool temperatures, and liquefies on contact with the skin. A nice combination.

⊛ EQUAL PARTS OF COCOA BUTTER, SESAME, AND MEADOWFOAM SEED OILS: makes a hard mixture but one that gives and liquefies quickly on the skin.

⊛ EQUAL PARTS OF KOKUM, BABASSU, AND SESAME OILS: makes a hard mix, gives with pressure and slowly dissolves on the skin.

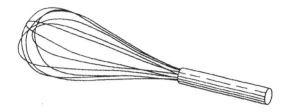

Whipped Body Butter

Description

These are delightful soft body butters that melt on contact when proportions are right. Combinations of saturated and unsaturated oils are combined, cooled, then whipped together with simple kitchen equipment to create light air-filled butters. If summer or ambient temperatures are too high, the mixtures can collapse and revert to their un-whipped state.

Ingredients:

Mango or babassu butter	4 oz
Coconut oil	4 oz
Shea butter, West African	2 ½ oz
Cocoa butter	1 ½ oz
Liquid oil, any mix (see suggestions below)	4 ½ oz

Directions:

Suggestions for the liquid oils to use in this mix include sunflower for economy, rosehip seed for nourishment and color, and grape-seed for balancing the saturated oils with toning properties. Melt all together, chill until the mixture is set, no longer liquid. This can be done in a refrigerator or overnight if temperatures are cool. When set, use a kitchen mixer or stick blender with whisk and whip. The longer that the mixture is whipped the lighter it will become. Essential oils can be added at any time.

Containers

This mixture must be spooned or ladled into wide-mouth jars. It is not pourable. Press the mixture into jars, using spatulas. Tamp jars down to release air pockets and fill to the brim. Cover with appropriate lids and wipe the outsides of the jars with rubbing alcohol and paper towels before applying labels.

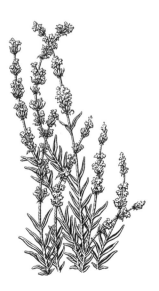

Oils and Herbs

Herbal oil infusions are time-tested combinations providing an amazing array of beneficial actions for the skin. By extracting beneficial botanical properties of leaves, flowers, stems, and roots into oil, the herb's phyto-medicinal properties are transferred to the oil for treatment of the skin and body.

INFUSING HERBS IN OIL

Infusing herbs into oil or fat is probably one of the oldest forms of medicine-making. Traditional methods in herbalism and perfumery use oils to extract scent and medicine. Submerging plant material in oil transfers the healing properties, scent, and color to the oil. Infusions of fresh or dried herbs transforms oil into a healing balm to be used directly or included in a cream or salve. The herbs used can be dried or fresh. However, plant material that has had all of its moisture removed through drying is easier to work with. If not handled correctly, moisture in fresh plant material can spoil your infusion.

Oil has a tendency to weep or wick; it will push out the top of the jar, especially in warm weather, and make a mess. Leave some room in the top of your infusing jars to allow for oil expansion and place a tray beneath your oil infusions to protect your counters or furniture.

WORKING WITH DRY HERBS

Place the plant material in a canning jar, filling it about a half to two-thirds full. Pour the oil over the plants and work the oil down into the dried material with a chopstick or skewer. Keep plant material submerged fully in the oil or it can develop mold where it is exposed to air. Placing a paper coffee filter cut to the size of the top of the jar, press the plant material down below the surface of the oil. The coffee filter will help trap the plant material below the surface of the oil and will protect your infusion. When submerged, pour more oil to cover the filter and plant material, leaving a bit of room for the oil to expand, and close with a lid.

WORKING WITH FRESH HERBS

I like to infuse fresh plants because, rightly or wrongly, I sense a life force that is still present in them. But fresh infusions need a bit of extra care and attention to avoid problems. When submerging fresh plant material into oil, the water contained in the leaves and flowers can overwhelm the oil with too much moisture and the infusion can go off or become moldy.

Pick your plant leaves or flowers early to mid-morning, on dry days when dew from the previous night has evaporated. Make sure there is no moisture on the leaves or flowers, picking only clean plant material and brushing off any dirt or insects. The plant material should not be washed before infusing. Wilting the aerial parts of plants by setting them aside in an open weave basket or colander for a day or overnight allows for some moisture to leave before infusing. When ready, place the plant parts in a jar (canning jars work well) and fill it to the top. Press the plants down some, but don't pack tightly. Pour oil over the plants, working it down into the material.

As with the dried herbs, keep plant material from poking out of the top of the oil by placing a paper coffee filter cut to the size of the top of the jar. Press the plant material down below the surface of the oil and filter, then top up with more oil to cover and close with a lid. Leave some room for the oil to expand in the jar.

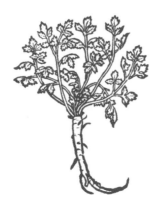

INFUSING FRESH ROOTS

Roots need to be washed free of mud and stones before infusing. When clean, lay them out on towels to air dry for several hours or overnight. The roots must be surface dry for a good infusion and to prevent mold growth. Cut the roots into smaller pieces and place in the jar. As with the plant tops, pour oil over the whole and seal, keeping plant material below the surface of the oil. Leave an inch or so at the top of the jar to make room for the oil's possible expansion.

TIME, SUN, AND HEAT: HOW TO INFUSE

Once plants are in the jar and oil poured over them, then what? The infusing process can take several forms; we will cover three of them here. Heat infusion is the fastest way to infuse, while cold infusing—letting the infusion proceed at its own pace—is the slowest. Solar infusing, using the powerful rays of the sun to imprint and create your herbal remedy, has its own benefits. Medicine-makers and herbalists use different methods based on their experience, location, and practice. Find the method that works best for you.

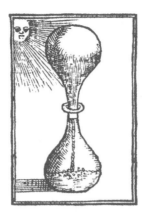

Sun infusion

Description

Placing herbs to be infused in the sun speeds the transfer of plant constituents and imprints the sun's energetic forces into the oil. Sun infusion is a method used by herbalists around the world to prepare St. John's Wort. While traditional for infusing that herb, any herb fresh or dried can be sun-infused. The sun's action on the plant material in the oil makes a special kind of energetic infusion.

Directions:

After filling the jars with either fresh or dry material and oil, place them outdoors to allow the sun's warmth and potent rays to assist in the transference of properties from plant to oil. Leave the jars for several days, up to a week. The length of time will depend on where you live. In the Pacific Northwest, I leave my jars for up to two weeks if the days are cool with scattered sun and clouds. In a very hot southern environment, I might leave the jars for only a few days.

Benefits:

The sun is a vital source of life. By using the sun's energy, the healing properties of the oil is heightened.

Plants to try:

St. John's Wort is the most traditional, but all plants can be sun infused; calendula, lavender, rosemary, lemon balm, yarrow, comfrey, roses, mugwort, violet leaves, lilac flowers, and elderflower are a few ideas

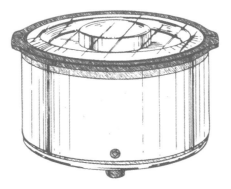

Heat infusion

Description

By using low heat, the infusion process is sped up. This process can be done in a crockpot or by low-heat oven method.

Directions:

Put the oil and herbs into the crockpot or pan. Leave temperature settings on very low heat for several hours. Watch the temperature with this method so that the oil doesn't overheat. It should remain in the range of 120 to 130 degrees. Too much heat will cause the infused oil to become rancid more quickly.

Benefits:

Infusing can be done in a concentrated period of time, and the oil then stored away for use in future products. The method provides an economy of time and attention.

Plants to try:

Any of the above plants can be infused by this method, dry or fresh. Also try with evergreen boughs, eucalyptus, jalapeno peppers, garlic, among others.

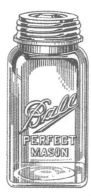
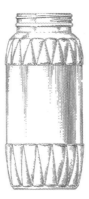

Cold infusion

Description

Time becomes the infusing action in this method and no additional heat is used. Jars of macerating oil can be left on a counter or in a cupboard while the transfer of phyto-chemicals from plant to oil occurs. Indoors, this can take up to six weeks or longer.

Directions:

Place herb and oil filled jars in a cupboard or on a counter where they can stay for up to six weeks or more. Place a tray under the jars to protect against oil weeping onto counters or down walls. Shake the jars from time to time to disperse the oil. Six weeks is the herbal standard and longer infusion times are not necessary.

Benefits:

The ease of this method is clear and there is a reduced likelihood of too much heat causing polyunsaturated oils, if used, to go rancid. The oils can sit for an extended period of time indoors, away from heat and light.

Plants to try:

Many plants with the exception of calendula can stay in the infusing oil for even longer periods; rose petals, St. John's Wort, rosemary, lavender. Some herbs however develop exceptionally strong odors that can interfere with future product making. Remove these herbs from the oil after the six week infusion period; calendula, lilac blossoms, plantain, comfrey are some of these.

WHICH OILS TO USE?

This book has covered a number of oils, but which one is best? This depends on what you want to achieve. If making salves or products, the longer shelf life the better. Cost is a factor too—infusing takes a lot of oil, some of which is lost in the process. End use and skin feel are other considerations. Most herbalists in the US use olive or pomace oil, as it is a fairly low-cost oil with a long shelf life. Older European traditions call for lard, the fat of pigs, as it is a stable, saturated fat and compatible with the skin. I find olive oil too oily for some of my products and switched from olive to sesame oil a number of years ago. At the time sesame oil was inexpensive (though that is no longer true), and it's as stable as olive oil. Sesame oil contains two natural preservatives, sesamin and sesamol, which help keep infusions for a good length of time when stored in the cool and dark. A note on sesame oil: sesame oil comes in two versions, unrefined and toasted. The toasted variety is strongly scented for Asian cooking and not usually used in skin care. Find the untoasted refined or unrefined type for making infusions.

Coconut oil can be used to extract scent from very aromatic flowers. A jasmine infusion turned out well by adding multiple rounds of flowers to the just-warmed oil over the period of a week. This is a form of DIY enfleurage that is very rewarding.

In general, oils high in omega-9 oleic acid are best for infusions. Oils like flax and hemp can go rancid quickly and take your herbal medicines with them. Omega-3 and 6 oils will not last long and the heat or time used to infuse will speed their oxidation process. Experiment on a small scale with pints or quarts to see which oil is best suited for your needs.

WHICH PLANTS ARE BEST?

Herbal books that can be used as points of reference abound. Here are a few suggestions to begin: evergreen trees, pines, spruce, firs, and eucalyptus create

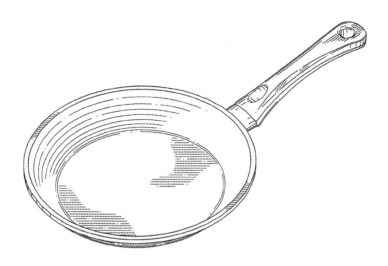

EQUIPMENT AND TOOLS

Gather and lay out before beginning:

※ A heavy pan—enameled cast iron are the best, or any heavy pan that spreads the heat over the surface and up the sides. Note: Pyrex can be difficult to use as the wax cools up the sides of the pan.

※ A heat source, such as a hot plate or stove. You will be keeping the temperatures low, so high heat is not necessary.

※ Spatulas, stirring sticks, or chopsticks (disposable chopsticks are useful and reusable).

※ Jars with lids.

※ Cleaning supplies, alcohol for jars and lids, paper towels, soap and water.

STEPS

Prepare the jars. Wash and dry them or disinfect your clean jars by wiping with some rubbing alcohol on a paper towel. Allow the rubbing alcohol to evaporate fully before filling. It dissipates quickly.

Measure the wax, place in the pan and gently melt over a low heat. Increase the heat slowly as needed and watch closely.

A note on temperature: Heat is the enemy of lipids and that includes oils, lecithin, and waxes. While we need heat to melt and combine the ingredients, keeping the temperature as low as possible preserves their structure. Oils and waxes should never get so hot that the mixture smokes. Harming your oils with excessive heat in the process of making products will shorten their life and make the oils turn rancid more quickly.

Back to the pan: As the wax melts, add the vegetable butter and keep melting slowly. When nearly melted, begin adding the liquid oils and heat only enough to re-melt the waxes. When adding cold oils, the wax will re-harden some. Keep melting slowly, stirring until the ingredients combine together homogeneously.

When the oils and waxes are fully melted it is time to add the essential oils. Gently stir them into the warm oil and wax mixture and mix thoroughly.

Testing the consistency: New recipes can have a lot of surprises. They can turn out too hard, too soft, or not set up at all! Believe me, you want to know that your recipe is right before pouring it into your jars. Luckily, this is easy to do. Drop a small amount of the warm mixture onto a clean saucer or piece of grease-proof paper and chill until set. Test the feel of the mix on hands or lips before pouring. Add more wax if it is too soft, or additional oil if too stiff, and test again.

Pouring: During the testing process, let the mix in the pan cool rather than keeping it hot and risking overheating. Reheat gently when you have the consistency you want and pour into the prepared small clean jars. Cover with a protective paper, letting the salve set in the jars.

Lids: When the salve is fully set the lids can be put on. Wipe away any dripped salve around the rim and down the sides of the jars with a paper towel and rubbing alcohol. The sides of the jars should remain clean and neat.

INGREDIENTS TO USE IN SALVES

Waxes: Beeswax thickens salves, lip balms, and solid perfumes beautifully. Warm on the skin, protective, pliable, and completely compatible with our skin, beeswax has been used throughout history—literally for millennia.

Beeswax can be purchased in blocks or in pastille form, as little pellets that are easy to measure. Measure them out ahead of time, since small pieces of wax are easiest to work with. A small scale is helpful but not necessary. Block wax needs to be made into smaller sizes so that it can be handled easily. It can be grated into smaller pieces, or use this method: melt thin layers of the wax off the block in the bottom of a heavy pan. As a layer cools, remove it from the pan and break into smaller pieces and store. Beeswax cools back to a solid quickly and in no time the block can be stored in pieces that are easy to handle.

Vegetable waxes generally have higher melting points than beeswax, making them more brittle, and recipes made with them are stiffer. Because of the higher melting point, the recipe will need less wax to achieve a similar consistency compared to one with beeswax.

Veganism avoids all animal products in any form and this includes beeswax. Vegetable waxes are therefore a must for products made for vegans. These waxes include candelilla, carnauba, rice bran, castor, and jojoba wax.

Some of these are natural waxes, and others made from hydrogenating the natural oils.

Essential oils for scent: Natural essential oils add therapeutic value as well as lovely aromas to body care. For a completely natural product, essential oils, rather than fragrance oils, are required. Essential oils can be added in different proportions. A 1+% dilution for an eight-ounce recipe is fifty drops essential oil. For a stronger scent, say for a solid perfume, 100 drops will bring the scent to a 2% dilution. Anything much greater than a 2% dilution can be overpowering to the senses for most products. With essential oils, less is often more.

Mixing essential oils is an art, and there are classes, books, and on line-courses that teach the basic principles. With time, favorite combinations and variations become second nature.

Lecithin is a phospholipid and useful for conditioning the skin. As a kind of lipid, it is very emollient and helps the skin take up and retain moisture. Adding it to a formula will increase the volume of wax needed to set the salve.

Vitamin E, a common antioxidant, helps keep oils from oxidizing and going rancid.

Basic proportions: an ounce of beeswax solidifies a cup, 8 ounces, of oil, to make a salve.

BUILDING A SALVE RECIPE OF YOUR OWN

Fixed oils: Vary the liquid oils that you use. Any liquid oil can be thickened with wax; try oils infused with plant materials or nutritious oils like rose hip seed, tamanu, evening primrose, or pomegranate. There is a nearly unlimited palette to choose from.

Vegetable butters and solid oils: Adding coconut oil, shea butter, cocoa butter, or any of the other tropical oils for some portion of the eight ounces of oil will add textural variety and additional healing properties and interest to the finished product. By including solid oils to the recipe, less beeswax or vegetable wax is necessary.

Extras: Clays, fruit powders, and herbal extracts can be mixed in for textural, color, or healing properties. Constant stirring while pouring combinations into jars keeps the suspended materials spread evenly. Clays and other solid powders will have a tendency to sink to the bottom of the pan if not kept stirred, giving the first few jars less and the last few more material.

Basic Salve Recipe

Description

This recipe makes a generous 8 ounces of salve. The ingredients are proportional, which means they can be varied as long as the ratio is preserved.

Ingredients:

Beeswax	1 oz
Liquid oil mixture	7 oz
Vegetable butter, shea, mango, etc.	1 oz
Essential oil	40 to 80 drops

Directions:

Gently begin melting beeswax and solid butters over low heat. When melted, add liquid oils slowly until the whole is melted and mixed together. Take care not to get the whole too hot. Add essential oils and mix again. Pour mixture into clean one, two, or four ounce jars. Let sit until set and put the lids on the jars. Label your creation.

ADDITIONAL IDEAS

- Add vitamin E to protect the oils and benefit the skin.

- Multiple oils can be used to make up the 8 ounces. If you add more solid oils, they should be a part of the 7 ounces. You may need less beeswax.

- For a solid lotion bar, use more saturated, solid oils and/or two to three ounces of beeswax.

- Cut the recipe in half and try variations.

- You can always re-melt everything and add more wax or more oil.

Lavender Salve

Description

Good for nerves or calming children, burns, wounds, or irritations, or just for the scent. Makes about 4 ounces or 120 ml of salve.

Ingredients:

Lavender infused oil *(or any high quality vegetable oil)*	½ cup or 4 ounces
Beeswax	½ oz, 1 tbs grated wax
Lavender essential oil	50 to 60 drops total

Directions:

Gently melt the beeswax, adding the lavender infused or plain oil slowly and mix together. When fully melted add the essential oil and stir in to combine all the ingredients. Once combined, pour the warm mixture into your prepared jars and allow to set. When the salve is cooled, cap the jars and clean the sides with rubbing alcohol so that labels will adhere to the jar

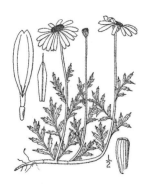

A Wild and Weedy Salve

Description

This is a good place to use the infused oils you have made and may not know what to do with! This salve is very healing, as it incorporates many herb combinations.

Ingredients:

Beeswax   1 ¼ oz
Shea or mango butter   2 oz
Infused oil   10 oz
(of a variety of infused oils, such as yarrow, calendula, St. John's Wort, comfrey)
Essential oils   80 drops
(of lavender, geranium, chamomile or other combination)

Directions:

Combine the beeswax and shea or mango butter in a heavy pan over low heat. When nearly melted, slowly add the oil portion, stirring to combine the whole mixture, then finish by adding the essential oils.

As you can see, there are many uses for the oils of the plant kingdom and we have only touched on a few of the basics. If you take nothing else away from this book know that oil is good; good for the skin and good for the body both inside and out. Eat oils, cook with the right ones, spread them on the body and bathe in their glory and familiarity with the cells of your body. Your whole being will welcome the nutritious compounds and reward you with good health.

APPENDICES

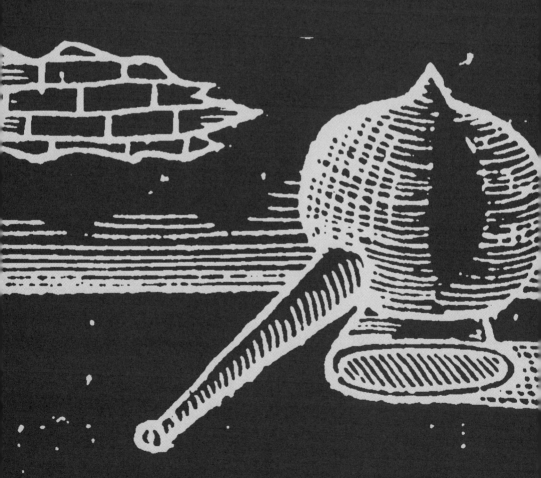

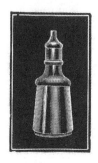

OILS BY USE

Vegetable Oils for Natural UV Protection

Avocado

Broccoli seed

Buriti

Carrot root & seed

Cherry kernel

Cranberry

Cucumber

Gevuina (Chilean hazelnut)

Hazelnut

Meadowfoam

Oat

Papaya

Red raspberry

Rice bran

Sesame

Shea butter

Tomato

Tropical oils in general

Yangu/Cape chestnut

Fading Skin Spots:

Avocado

Castor oil

Papaya

Rice bran

Rosehip seed

Acne, Psoriasis, Eczema:

Andiroba

Argan

Chia

Kukui

Nigella

Perilla

Sacha inchi

Anti-Aging:

Andiroba

Argan

Avocado

Blackberry

Buriti

Calophyllum

inophyllum (Tamanu)

Camelina

Camellia

Carrot seed

Cranberry

Cucumber

Gevuina (Chilean hazelnut)

Macadamia

Marula

Moringa

Oat

Passion fruit

Pomegranate

Sacha inchi

Tomato

Muscular Aches & Swellings:

Andiroba

Argan

Black currant

Nigella

Papaya

Passion fruit

Pomegranate

Shea Butter

Hair Care:

Abyssinian

Broccoli seed

Camellia tea oil

Carrot seed oil

Pequi

Scarring & Stretch Marks:

Buriti

Camellia

Chia

Cocoa Butter

Coconut

Cucumber

Rosehip seed oil

Massage:

Almond

Apricot kernel

Avocado

Coconut

Jojoba

Kukui

Macadamia

Olive

Sesame

Shea oil

Sunflower

To Help Preserve Products:

Baobab

Marula

Meadowfoam

Moringa

Watermelon

Traditional Medicinal Oils:

Andiroba

Castor oil

Caulophyllum

inophyllum (Tamanu)

Neem

Nigella

Shea

Wound Care:

Andiroba	Perilla
Caulophyllum	Pracaxi
inophyllum (Tamanu)	Pumpkin seed
Karanj	Rosehip seed
Kukui	
Neem	
Nigella	

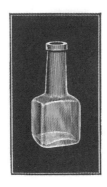

OILS BY PROPERTIES

Drying Oils:

Flax/Linseed   Poppy seed

Hemp seed   Walnut

Hi-Linoleic Safflower

Hi-Linoleic Sunflower

Perilla

Astringent Oils, High in Tannins, Dry Oils:

Camellia   Mango butter

Cranberry seed   Rose hip seed

Grape-seed

Hazelnut

Jojoba

Oils High in Stable Forms of Vitamin C:

Black Currant

Blackberry

Blueberry

Buriti

Kiwi seed

Marula

Passion fruit

Rose hip seed

Sea buckthorn

Oils High in Squalene:

Argan

Camellia

Gevuina (Chilean hazelnut)

Macadamia

Olive

Rice Bran

Wheat Germ

Oils with High Phospholipid Content:

Avocado

Kiwi seed

Marula

Oat

Poppy seed

Soybean

Oils Very High in Oleic Acid *(Omega-9, over 60%)*:

Acai	60%
Almond	65%
Apricot kernel	65%
Avocado	70%
Buriti	80%
Camellia	80%
Carrot Seed	68%
Hazelnut	80%
Macadamia Nut	60%
Marula	75%
Moringa	70%
Olive	75%
Papaya	70%
Peach kernel	60%
Plum kernel	70%
Shea oil	70%
Hi-Oleic Safflower	75%
Hi-Oleic Sunflower	72%

Oils Moderate in Oleic Acid *(Omega-9, 35–59%)*:

Andiroba	50%
Argan	45%
Baobab	35%
Brazil nut	45%
Calophyllum inophyllum (Tamanu)	49%
Canola	58%
Cocoa butter	35%
Gevuina (Chilean hazelnut)	50%

Karanj	55%
Kokum butter	35%
Mango butter	48%
Neem	50%
Oat seed	40%
Palm	40%
Peanut	45%
Pecan	52%
Pequi	50%
Pistachio	53%
Pracaxi	55%
Rice bran	35%
Sal butter	45%
Sesame	45%
Shea Butter	48%
Yangu	45%

Oils with Significant Linoleic Acid *(Omega-6, 50%+)*:

Acai	50%
Blackberry seed	60%
Cucumber	65%
Evening primrose	70%
Grape-seed	76%
Hemp	55%
Milk Thistle	55%
Nigella	58%
Passion fruit seed	75%
Poppy seed	70%
Pumpkin seed	55%

Red Raspberry	50%
Safflower	75%
Soybean	50%
Sunflower	72%
Tomato seed	55%
Walnut	55%
Watermelon	60%
Wheat germ	55%

Oils with Moderate Linoleic Acid *(Omega-6, 30–49%)*:

Argan	45%
Baobab	35%
Black currant	47%
Blueberry	45%
Borage	35%
Brazil nut	45%
Cherry kernel	44%
Coffee bean, green	40%
Corn	48%
Cranberry	40%
Kukui	40%
Oat seed	40%
Peach kernel	30%
Peanut	33%
Pecan	36%
Pistachio	34%
Rice bran	40%
Rose hip seed	45%
Sacha Inchi	35%

Sea Buckthorn	35%
Sesame	40%
Soybean	50%

Oils with Significant Alpha-Linolenic Acid *(Omega-3, 15%+)*:

Blackberry	15%
Blueberry	28%
Camelina	45%
Chia seed	60%
Cranberry	30%
Flax	65%
Hemp	20%
Kiwi seed	58%
Kukui nut	35%
Perilla	55%
Red raspberry	22%
Rose hip seed	35%
Sacha inchi	48%
Sea buckthorn	32%
Walnut	15%

Oils with Significant Palmitoleic Acid:

Avocado	13%
Gevuina (Chilean hazelnut)	25%
Macadamia nut	20%
Sea buckthorn fruit	24%

Omega-3 to Omega-6 Ratios of Significance:

| Blueberry | 1:1.5 |
| Camelina | 2:1 |

Chia seed	3:1
Cranberry seed	1:1
Flax	2:1
Hemp	1:3
Kiwi	3:1
Kukui	1:1.5
Perilla	3:1
Red raspberry	1:2
Rose hip seed	1:1
Sacha inchi	1: 0.7
Sea Buckthorn seed	1:1

Oils with Very-Long-Chain Fatty Acids:

Abyssinian

Broccoli seed

Meadowfoam

Daikon radish

Jojoba

Oils with Significant Gamma-Linolenic Acid *(Omega-6)*:

Black currant	17%
Borage seed	25%
Evening primrose	10%

Oils High in Lauric Acid, Medium-Chain Fatty Acids:

Coconut	50%
Babassu	47%
Palm Kernel	48%

+ many new tropical butters

Oils with Significant Erucic Acid:

Abyssinian	60%
Broccoli seed	49%
Daikon radish seed	34%
Jojoba oil	18%
Meadowfoam	13%

Oils with High Unsaponifiable Content:

Avocado

Mango butter

Nilotica shea

Rice Bran

Shea butter

Wheat germ

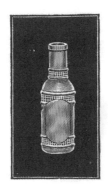

OILS BY SOURCE

The Tropical Oils:

Acai	Mango
Babassu	Palm variations
Brazil nut	Papaya
Buriti	Pequi
Cocoa butter	Shea butter & oil
Coconut	

Dry Climate Oils, Halophytes:

Argan	Watermelon seed
Baobab	Yangu
Jojoba	

Oils from Kernels:

Acai	Mango
Almond	Palm kernels
Apricot	Peach
Cherry	Plum

Oils from Beans/Legumes:

Castor   Peanut

Cocoa   Pracaxi

Coffee   Soy

Karanj

Oils from Grains/Grasses:

Oat   Rice bran

Corn

Wheat germ

Oils from Seeds

Abyssinian   Milk thistle

Black currant   Nigella

Blackberry   Oat

Blueberry   Papaya seed

Borage   Passion fruit seed

Broccoli seed   Perilla

Camelina   Pomegranate

Camellia, tea seed   Poppy

Carrot seed   Pumpkin

Chia   Raspberry

Cranberry   Rosehip seed

Cucumber   Safflower

Daikon radish   Sesame

Evening primrose   Sunflower

Flax   Tomato

Grape-seed   Watermelon

Kiwi seed   Wheat germ

Meadowfoam

Oils From Fruiting Bodies *(Often Results in Two Sources Of Oil)*

Avocado

Olives

Palm

Pracaxi

Sea buckthorn

Oils from Ancient Food & Oil Crops

Camelina

Castor

Flax

Hemp

Moringa

Nigella

Olive

Safflower

Sesame

Watermelon

Oils from Africa

Argan

Baobab

Marula

Moringa

Palm

Shea

Shea Nilotica

Watermelon, Ootanga

Yangu

Oils from South America

Acai

Andiroba

Babassu

Brazil nut

Buriti

Gevuina (Chilean

hazelnut)

Passion fruit

Pequi

Pracaxi

Rosehip

Sacha inchi

Oils from the Pacific

Caulophyllum	Kiwi
inophyllum	Kukui
Cocoa butter	Macadamia
Coconut	Mango
Illipe	Papaya

Oils from the Middle East & Mediterranean

Abyssinian	Olive
Almond	Pomegranate
Apricot	Poppy
Nigella	

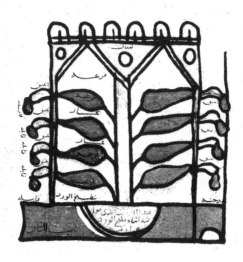

BOTANICAL FAMILIES OF
OIL-BEARING PLANTS

Plants are classed into groups according to their similarities and shared qualities. Taxonomy is the discipline of grouping according to *taxa*, plural, or *taxon*, singular, into units of similar properties. Carolus Linnaeus, the Swedish botanist, is famous for trying to bring order and relationships to the wide diversity of plant, animal, and mineral life forms. He published his classifications in 1758, and they are still in use today.

The kingdom *Plantae* includes the plant oils. Under "kingdom" falls the classification "order," and then "family." Next after family is "genus," and finally "species," where the greatest diversity is catalogued.

Plant families share characteristics among their members, creating a picture or family snapshot that can help the understanding of qualities or properties. Of the oil-bearing plants, the cabbage (*Brassica*) family has a number of members with a particular fatty acid profile. The grasses, *Poaceae*, produce nourishing oils. The major food-bearing family rose, *Rosaceae*, has a number of fruit, seeds, and kernels that are pressed for oil.

Understanding plant families helps link relationships that may shed light on beneficial or cautionary use of the plants. For example, both castor and kukui nut are members of the same family, *Euphorbiaceae,* and both have properties that make them indigestible but useful for treating the skin.

Anacardiaceae

Mango Butter
Marula
Pistachio

Actinidiaceae

Kiwi

Arecaceae / Palmae / Palm

Acai
Babassu
Buriti
Coconut
Palm oil
Palm Kernel oil

Asteraceae/ Daisy

Safflower
Sunflower
Milk thistle seed

Bombacaceae

Baobab

Boraginaceae

Borage seed

Brassicaceae / Cabbage

Abyssinian

Broccoli seed
Camelina
Canola/Rapeseed
Daikon radish seed

Calophyllaceae / St John's Wort Family

Tamanu, Foraha, *Caulophyllum inophyllum*

Cannabaceae

Hemp seed

Caricaeae

Papaya

Caryocaraceae

Pequi

Corylaceae / Betulaceae

Hazelnut

Cucurbitaceae / Gourd

Cucumber seed
Pumpkin seed
Watermelon seed

Euphorbiaceae

Castor oil
Kukui nut
Sacha inchi

Dipterocarpaceae

Illipe butter

Elaeagnaceae

Sea buckthorn

Ericaceae / Vaccinium

> Cranberry
> Blueberry

Fabaceae / Legumes

> Karanj
> Peanut
> Pracaxi
> Soybean

Grossulariaceae / Ribes / Currant

> Black currant

Juglandaceae

> Walnut
> Pecan

Lamiaceae / Mint

> Perilla
> Chia

Lauraceae / Laurel

> Avocado

Lecythidaceae

> Brazil nut

Limnanthaceae

> Meadowfoam seed

Linaceae / Linum

> Flax

Lythraceae

    Pomegranate

Malvaceae

    Cocoa butter

Meliaceae

    Neem
    Andiroba

Moringaceae / Horseradish tree family

    Moringa

Oleaceae

    Olive

Onagraceae

    Evening Primrose

Papaveraceae / Poppy

    Poppy

Passifloraceae

    Passion fruit

Pedaliaceae

    Sesame

Poaceae/ Grasses

    Corn
    Oat
    Rice Bran
    Wheat germ

Proteaceae

> Macadamia
> Gevuina (Chilean hazelnut)

Ranunculaceae

> Black seed/Nigella

Rosaceae / Rose

> Almond
> Apricot kernel
> Blackberry Seed
> Cherry kernel
> Peach kernel
> Plum kernel
> Raspberry
> Rose hip seed

Rubiaceae

> Coffee

Rutaceae

> Cape Chestnut, Yangu

Sapotaceae

> Argan
> Nilotica shea
> Shea butter
> Shea oil

Simmondsiaceae

> Jojoba

Solanaceae

> Tomato seed

Theaceae / Tea

Camellia

Umbelliferae / *Apiaceae* / Carrot

Carrot seed
Carrot root

Vitaceae

Grape-seed

SAPONIFICATION VALUES
FOR 90 OILS, FATS, AND WAXES

Abyssinian	167
Acai	191
Almond	192.5
Andiroba	186
Apricot kernel	190.0
Argan	189
Avocado	187.5
Babassu	247.0
Beef tallow	197.0
Black currant	188
Blackberry	189.5
Blueberry	190
Borage seed	188.0
Brazil nut	245.0
Broccoli seed	200
Buriti	210
Butterfat, cow	226.6
Camelina	185.9
Camellia	191
Canola oil/Rapeseed	174.7
Castor	180.3*
Caulophyllum Inophyllum	208
Cherry kernel	190
Chia seed	191.5
Cocoa butter	193.8
Coconut	268.0
Coffee, green	193
Coffee, roasted	186
Corn	192.0
Cranberry	190
Cucumber	183

Daikon radish seed	176
Emu oil	195.0
Evening primrose	191.0
Flax seed/Linseed	189.9
Goat tallow	193.6
Goose fat	191.6
Grape-seed	182.5
Hazelnut	195.0
Hemp seed	192.8
Illipe butter	192.5
Jojoba	97.5
Karanj	183
Kiwi seed	196
Kokum butter	189.4
Kukui nut	190.0
Lanolin	103.7
Lard	194.6
Macadamia nut	195.0
Mango butter	194.8
Marula	190
Meadowfoam	169
Milk thistle	196
Moringa	195
Neem	194.5
Nigella	193
Nutmeg butter	162.4
Oat	190
Olive	189.7
Palm	199.1
Palm kernel	219.9
Papaya	188
Passion fruit	193
Perilla	191
Pistachio nut	191.0
Pomace/Olive	189.7
Pomegranate	190

Poppy seed	193.6
Pracaxi	180
Pumpkin seed	193.0
Red raspberry	186
Rice bran	179.2
Rose hip seed	193.0
Safflower	192.0
Sal butter	190.0
Sea buckthorn	163
Sesame	187.9
Shea butter	180.0
Sheep tallow	193.6
Soybean oil/shortening	190.6
Sunflower seed	188.7
Tomato seed	192
Walnut	189.4
Watermelon seed	191.5
Wheat germ	185.0
Yangu/Cape chestnut	190

Waxes

Beeswax	88–100
Candelilla wax	44–66
Carnauba wax	78–95
Jojoba wax	85–95

* Due to castor oil's unusual fatty acid composition, it doesn't behave like other oils with its SAP value. Generally its percentage in soap should be not more than 10 to 15%.

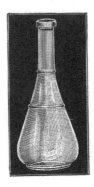

FATTY ACID FAMILIES OF OILS

Oils and fats fall into families characterized by the degree of saturation of the oils in the group. The following is a brief description of each oil family.

The "omega" designation is determined by the number of carbon atoms from the free end, the omega end, of the fatty acid to the first double bond. The first double bond occurs at the third carbon atom in an omega-3 fatty acid. In an omega-9 monounsaturated oil, it occurs at the ninth carbon atom.

☀ **Super-Unsaturated, Omega-3 Family:** the most unsaturated, with three double bonds. It includes the essential alpha-Linolenic acid (18:3), LNA, of which flax seed oil is the highest vegetable source. This group also contains stearidonic acid (18:4), SDA, found in black currant seed oil, as well as eicosapentaenoic (20:5) acid, EPA, and docosahexaenoic acid (22:6), DHA, which are found in cold-water fish and marine animals.

☀ **Super-Unsaturated, Omega-5 Family:** includes punicic acid (18:3), from pomegranate, a highly nutritious, long-chain fatty acid with 18 carbons that is super-unsaturated with three conjugated double bonds. Monounsaturated myristoleic acid from nutmeg and eleostearic acid found in cherry kernels are also of this family.

⊛ **Polyunsaturated, Omega-6 Family**: has two double bonds and includes the essential linoleic acid, LA, found in safflower, sunflower, hemp, soybean, walnut, and sesame oils. Also included in this group is gamma-Linolenic acid, GLA, found in borage, black currant seed, and evening primrose oil. Arachidonic acid, AA, found in meats and other animal products, and dihomo-gamma-linolenic acid (DGLA), found in human breast milk, is also included here.

⊛ **Monounsaturated, Omega-7 Family**: represented by palmitoleic acid, POA, which is found in tropical oils such as coconut and palm kernel. It has one double bond in a 16-carbon fatty acid chain (16:1). Vaccenic acid (18:1) named from the Latin for cow, *vacca*, is found in dairy sources, including milk, butter, and human breast milk. A version, cis-vaccenic acid, is also found in Sea Buckthorn oil.

⊛ **Monounsaturated, Omega-8 Family**: one representative of this family is the rare margaroleic acid (17:1), which is found in fish and animal fats primarily and occasionally in plant oils.

⊛ **Monounsaturated, Omega-9 Family**: Mono means one double bond in the 18-carbon fatty acid chain. This major family is represented by oleic acid, OA, (18:1), a fatty acid found in large quantities in many oils: olive, avocado, almond, macadamia nut, pecan, and peanut oil are a few. Erucic acid is a long-chain fatty acid with a 22-carbon chain, but only one double bond (22:1).

⊛ **Saturated Family**: includes stearic acid, SA, found in red meat, butter, cocoa butter, and shea butter; palmitic acid, PA, found in tropical fats; butyric acid, BA, found in butter; and arachidic acid, found in peanuts.

LISTING OF COMMON FATTY ACIDS BY SATURATION AND OMEGA FAMILY

The Saturated Fatty Acids

The list below groups common fatty acids by their saturation level and omega family, and includes the shorthand name and primary sources for each type of fatty acid.

Short-Chain Saturated Fatty Acid

Butyric Acid (C4:0)	Dairy
Caproic Acid (C6:0)	Dairy, goats

Medium-Chain Saturated Fatty Acid

Caprylic Acid (C8:0)	Dairy milk, coconut
Capric Acid (C10:0)	Milk, coconut, palm kernel
Lauric Acid (C12:0)	Coconut

Long-Chain Saturated Fatty Acid

Myristic Acid (C14:0)	Nutmeg butter
Pentadecanoic Acid (C15:0)	Dairy
Palmitic Acid (C16:0)	Fish, Dairy, Plant
Margaric Acid (C17:0)	Goat milk, rare
(also known as heptadecanoic acid)	
Stearic Acid (C18:0)	Animal, vegetable fats
Arachidic Acid (C20:0)	Peanut oil
(also known as icosanoic acid or eicosanoic acid)	

Very-Long-Chain Saturated Fatty Acid

Behenic Acid (C22:0)   Plant, peanut, others

Lignoceric Acid (C24:0)   Plant, peanut

Cerotic Acid (C26:0)   Beeswax, carnauba wax

The Unsaturated Fatty Acids

We've discussed metabolites and isomers that are the chemistry lab of our bodies, molecules created from the foods we eat that provide for the complex functioning of the body. One such group of molecules is the eicosanoids (the IUPAC name is icosanoids), messenger molecules made when 20 carbon fatty acid chains are oxidized. These molecules control many body functions, including inflammation and immunity. The extent and complexity is vast and not our subject here, except to say that it produces a dizzying array of fatty acids with the same name or nearly the same names. Eicosenoic acid, C20:1, comes in three omega varieties; move the double bond and, voila, three different fatty acids appear: omega 7, omega 9, and omega 11, all 20 carbon monounsaturated fatty acids. Other fatty acid groups share the name octadecatrienoic but have different levels of unsaturation. So consider this a heads up that the proper names for fatty acids can be confusing.

Monounsaturated Fatty Acids Omega 11

Gondoic/Eicosenoic Acid (C20:1)   Marine, cod liver, whale oils

Unsaturated Fatty Acids, Omega-10

Sapienic Acid (16:1)   Human only

Sabaleic Acid (18:2)   Human only

(Precious little information exists for sabaleic acid, but I've left it in the list as new research may show it to be more important.)

Monounsaturated Fatty Acids, Omega-9

Oleic Acid (C18:1)	Plant, animal fat
Ricinoleic Acid (C18:1)	Castor beans
Gadoleic/Eicosenoic Acid (C20:1)	Cabbage, cod, and whale oils
Erucic/Docosenoic Acid (C22:1)	Seed oils, various
Nervonic Acid (C24:1)	Shark liver

Monounsaturated Fatty Acids, Omega-8

Margaroleic Acid (C17:1)	Primarily Marine

(Also known as heptadecenoic Acid)

Monounsaturated Fatty Acids, Omega-7

Palmitoleic Acid, POA (C16:1)	Animal, plant, marine

(Also known as hexadecenoic acid)

Vaccenic Acid (C18:1)	Dairy, animal fat
Paullinic/Eicosenoic Acid (C20:1)	Herring oil, rapeseed

Polyunsaturated Fatty Acids, Omega-6

Linoleic Acid, LA (C18:2)	Seed, nut oils
Gamma-Linolenic Acid, GLA (C18:3)	Black Currant, animal
Eleostearic Acid (C18:3)	Cherry kernel
Eicosadienoic Acid, EDA (C20:2)	Animal, marine
Dihomo-gamma-linolenic Acid, DGLA (C20:3)	Trace amounts, rare
Arachidonic Acid, AA (C20:4)	Peanut, animal, egg

(Also known as eicosatetraenoic acid)

Brassic/Docosadienoic Acid (C22:2)	rare

Polyunsaturated Fatty Acids, Omega 5

Eleostearic Acid (C18:3)   Cherry kernel
(Also called octadecatrienoic acid)
Punicic Acid (C18:3)   Pomegranate
Myristoleic Acid (C14:1)   Nutmeg

Superunsaturated Fatty Acid, Omega-3

Alpha-Linolenic Acid LNA (C18:3)   Plants; flax, hemp
Stearidonic Acid SDA (C18:4)   Hemp, black currant
Eicosatetraenoic Acid ETA (C20:4)   Shark liver, herring
Timnodonic Acid EPA (C20:5)   Marine, animal
(Also called Eicosapentaenoic Acid)
Clupanodonic Acid DPA (C22:5)   Animal liver, herring
(Also called Docosapentaenoic Acid)
Cervonic Acid DHA (C22:6)   Marine, plant
(Also called Docosahexaenoic Acid)

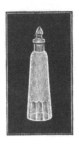

FATTY ACID TABLES AND COMPOSITION FOR THE OILS

These tables have been culled from a wide number of sources, including supplier data sheets, research papers, and internet articles. For this reason, the formats vary, and the information on some oils is more complete than on others.

The fatty acid composition of oils is never absolute. It varies depending on a host of factors, including growing conditions, region, plant variety, and other characteristics. View the fatty acid information as indicative of each oil rather than definitive.

The fatty acid patterns and composition help us understand the properties of oils. Comparing oils to one another must begin with the fatty acids, as they are the majority of the oil. A quick glance at a fatty acid table will bring its oils' dominant qualities into focus. The balance between the different fatty acids, long and short, saturated or not, contribute considerably to the feel, function, and action of the oil as a whole.

All oils have an unsaponifiable portion, and this information is readily available for some oils and not others. The fatty acids are listed by percentage of the oil, from the greatest to trace amounts.

Note: We've reviewed many fatty acids, many of which you will know at this point in the book. The more unusual fatty acids are coded here for your convenience. For example, 22:1 is the code for erucic acid, a 20 carbon chain with one double bond.

A reminder:
> greater than
< less than

ABYSSINIAN OIL

Erucic Acid	50–65%	C22:1
Oleic Acid	10–25%	
Linoleic Acid	7–15%	
Eicosenoic Acid	2–6%	C20:1
Alpha-Linolenic Acid	2–5%	
Palmitic Acid	1–4%	
Behenic Acid	1–3%	C22:0
Stearic Acid	0.5–2%	
Arachidic Acid	0.5–2%	C20:1
Eicosadienoic Acid	0–4%	C20:2
Lignoceric Acid	0–1%	C24:0
Palmitoleic Acid	0.1–0.5%	C16:1

ACAI OIL

Oleic Acid	60%	
Linoleic Acid	50%	
Palmitic Acid	18%	
Stearic Acid	1.5%	
Alpha-Linolenic Acid	1.5%	
Lauric Acid	trace%	C12:0
Palmitoleic Acid	trace%	C16:1

ALMOND OIL (SWEET)

Oleic Acid	60–75%	
Linoleic Acid	20–30%	
Palmitic Acid	3–9%	
Stearic Acid	0.5–3%	
Alpha-Linolenic Acid	0.4%	
Arachidic Acid	0.2%	C20:0

Eicosenoic Acid	0.2%	C20:1
Behenic Acid	0.2%	C22:0
Erucic Acid	0.1%	C22:1
Unsaponifiables	<1.5%	

ANDIROBA OIL

Oleic Acid	50.5%	
Palmitic Acid	28%	
Linoleic Acid	11%	
Stearic Acid	8.1%	
Arachidic Acid	1.2%	C20:0
Palmitoleic Acid	1%	C16:1
Alpha-Linolenic Acid	1.3%	
Behenic	0.34%	C22:0
Myristic Acid	0.33%	C14:0
Unsaponifiables	3–5%	

APRICOT KERNEL OIL

Oleic Acid	55–74%	
Linoleic Acid	20–35%	
Palmitic Acid	3–7%	
Stearic Acidtrace	–2%	
Palmitoleic Acidtrace	–1.4%	C16:1
Alpha-Linolenic Acidtrace	–1%	
Eicosenoic Acidtrace	–1%	C20:1
Unsaponifiables	0.5–0.7%	

ARGAN OIL

Oleic Acid	45–47%	

Linoleic Acid	31–35%	
Palmitic Acid	12–14%	
Stearic Acid	5.5–5.7%	
Alpha-Linolenic Acid	0.5%	
Eicosenoic Acid	0.5%	C20:1
Arachidic Acid	0.4%	C20:0
Myristic Acid	0.2%	C14:0
Unsaponifiables	<1%	

AVOCADO OIL

Oleic Acid	50–80%	
Palmitic Acid	12–20%	
Linoleic Acid	6–18%	
Palmitoleic Acid	2–13%	C16:1
Alpha-Linolenic Acid	5% max.	
Stearic Acid	1–2%	
Unsaponifiables	2–11%	

BABASSU OIL

Lauric Acid	47.3%	C12:0
Myristic Acid	14.5%	C14:0
Oleic Acid	12.2%	
Capric Acid	8.3%	C10:0
Caprylic Acid	7.1%	C8:0
Palmitic Acid	7.1%	C16:0
Stearic Acid	2.0%	
Linoleic Acid	1.1%	
Caproic Acid	0.3%	C6:0

BAOBAB OIL

Oleic Acid	30–40%
Linoleic Acid	24–34%
Palmitic Acid	18–30%
Stearic Acid	2–8%
Alpha-Linolenic Acid	1–3%

BLACKBERRY SEED OIL

Linoleic Acid	63.2%
Alpha-Linolenic Acid	15.2%
Oleic Acid	15.1%
Palmitic Acid	3.4%
Stearic Acid	2.1%

BLACK CURRANT OIL

Linoleic Acid	47–48%	
Gamma-Linolenic Acid	16–17%	C18:3
Oleic Acid	9–11%	
Palmitic Acid	6%	
Stearidonic Acid	2.5–3.5%	C18:4
Stearic Acid	1.5%	
Unsaponifiables	<4%	

BLUEBERRY SEED OIL

Linoleic Acid	40–45%	
Alpha-Linolenic Acid	25–30%	
Oleic Acid	18–22%	
Palmitic Acid	3–6%	
Stearic Acid	1–3%	
Arachidic Acid	1%	C20:0

Eicosenoic Acid	0–.4%	C20:1
Behenic Acid	0.3%	C22:0
Palmitoleic Acid	0.1%	C16:1
Myristic Acid	0.1%	C14:0

BORAGE SEED OIL

Linoleic Acid	35–40%	
Gamma-Linolenic Acid	20–28%	C18:3
Oleic Acid	15–20%	
Palmitic Acid	9–12%	
Stearic Acid	3–5%	
Eicosenoic Acid	3–5%	C20:1
Erucic Acid	2–3%	C22:1
Nervonic Acid	1–2%	C24:1
Unsaponifiables	1–2%	

BRAZIL NUT OIL

Oleic Acid	35–50%	
Linoleic Acid	25–40 %	
Palmitic Acid	15–28%	
Stearic Acid	6–9%	
Arachidic Acid	1–1.5%	C20:0
Palmitoleic Acid	0.5–1%	C16:1
Myristic Acid	0.2–0.6%	C14:0
Alpha-Linolenic Acid	0.1–0.3%	

BROCCOLI SEED OIL

Erucic Acid	49%	C22:1
Oleic Acid	13.5%	
Linoleic Acid	11.4%	

Alpha-Linolenic Acid	9%	
Eicosenoic Acid	6%	C20:1
Palmitic Acid	3.25%	C16:0

BURITI OIL

Oleic Acid	79.2%	
Palmitic Acid	16.3%	
Linoleic Acid	1.4%	
Alpha-Linolenic Acid	1.3%	
Stearic Acid	1.3%	
Palmitoleic Acid	0.4%	C16:1

CAMELINA OIL

Alpha-Linolenic Acid	38–45%	
Linoleic Acid	22%	
Oleic Acid	16.7%	
Eicosenoic Acid	16.1%	C20:1
Palmitic Acid	6.5%	
Stearic Acid	2.2%	
Erucic Acid	2%	C22:1
Palmitoleic Acid	<1	C16:1
Myristic Acid	<1	C14:0

CAMELLIA SEED OIL

Oleic Acid	80%	
Linoleic Acid	9%	
Palmitic Acid	9%	
Stearic Acid	1%	
Arachidic Acid	1%	C20:0

CANOLA OIL

Oleic Acid	56–62%	
Linoleic Acid	21–28%	
Alpha-Linolenic Acid	8–13%	
Palmitic Acid	3–5%	
Stearic Acid	1.3–1.7%	
Erucic Acid	2%	C22:1
Palmitoleic Acid	0.2–0.3%	C16:1

CARROT SEED OIL

Oleic Acid	68%
Linoleic Acid	10.8
Stearic Acid	7%
Palmitic Acid	3.7%
Alpha-Linolenic Acid	0.2%

CASTOR OIL

Ricinoleic Acid	90%	C18:1
Linoleic Acid	5–7%	
Oleic Acid	3–7%	
Palmitic Acid	1–2%	
Stearic Acid	<1.5%	
Alpha-Linolenic Acid	<0.5%	
Unsaponifiables	0.5–1%	

CAULOPHYLLUM INOPHYLLUM/TAMANU OIL

Oleic Acid	49%
Linoleic Acid	21.3%
Palmitic Acid	14.7%

Stearic Acid	12.6%	
Myristic Acid	2.5%	C14:0
Alpha-Linolenic Acid	<0.5%	
Eicosanoic Acid	0.94%	C20:1
Calophyllic Acid (unique to this oil)		

CHERRY KERNEL OIL

Linoleic Acid	44%	
Oleic Acid	32%	
Eleostearic Acid	12%	C18:3
Palmitic Acid	7.5%	
Stearic Acid	2.1%	
Arachidic Acid	1.1%	C20:0
Alpha-Linolenic Acid	1%	
Palmitoleic Acid	0.5%	C16:1
Eicosenoic Acid	0.4%	C20:1

CHIA SEED OIL

Alpha-Linolenic Acid	59%
Linoleic Acid	21%
Oleic Acid	8.7%
Palmitic Acid	7%
Stearic Acid	2.1%

COCOA BUTTER

Oleic Acid	34–36%
Stearic Acid	31–35%
Palmitic Acid	25–30%
Linoleic Acid	approx. 3%
Unsaponifiables	<0.8%

COCONUT OIL

Lauric Acid	39–54%	C12:0
Myristic Acid	15–23%	C14:0
Caprylic Acid	6–10%	C8:0
Palmitic Acid	6–11%	C16:0
Capric Acid	5–10%	C10:0
Oleic Acid	4–11%	
Stearic Acid	1–4%	
Linoleic Acid	1–2%	
Unsaponifiables	0.6–1.5%	

CORN OIL

Linoleic Acid	46–56%
Oleic Acid	28–37%
Palmitic Acid	12–14%
Stearic Acid	2.3–2.7%
Unsaponifiables	1–2%

COFFEE OIL, Green

Palmitic Acid	40%	
Linoleic Acid	38 %	
Oleic Acid	8%	
Stearic Acid	8%	
Alpha-Linolenic Acid	2%	
Behenic Acid	1%	C22:0
Palmitoleic Acid	0.4%	C16:1

CRANBERRY SEED OIL

Linoleic Acid	35–45%
Alpha-Linolenic Acid	22–35%

Oleic Acid	20–25%	
Palmitic Acid	3–6%	
Stearic Acid	0.5–2%	
Palmitoleic Acid	0.5%	
Arachidic Acid	<1	C20:0
Tetraenoic Acid	<1	C20:4

CUCUMBER SEED OIL

Linoleic Acid	60–68%
Oleic Acid	14–20%
Palmitic Acid	9–13%
Stearic Acid	6–9%
Alpha-Linolenic Acid	<1%

DAIKON RADISH SEED OIL

Erucic Acid	34%	C22:1
Oleic Acid	20%	
Gadoleic Acid	10%	C20:1
Alpha-Linolenic Acid	12%	
Linoleic Acid	10%	
Palmitic Acid	4%	

EVENING PRIMROSE OIL

Linoleic Acid	65–75%	
Gamma-Linolenic Acid	9–11%	C18:3
Oleic Acid	5–11%	
Palmitic Acid	5–8%	
Stearic Acid	1–3%	
Arachidic Acid	2% max	C20:0

Eicosenoic Acid	2% max	C20:1
Alpha-Linolenic Acid	0.5%	

FLAX SEED OIL

Alpha-Linolenic Acid	35–66%
Oleic Acid	14–39%
Linoleic Acid	7–19%
Palmitic Acid	4–9%
Stearic Acid	2–4%
Unsaponifiables	0.5–1%

GEVUINA (CHILEAN HAZELNUT)

Oleic Acid	40–55%
Palmitoleic Acid	20–27%
Linoleic Acid	6–15%
Alpha-Linolenic Acid	2%

GRAPE-SEED OIL

Linoleic Acid	69–78%	
Oleic Acid	15–25 %	
Palmitic Acid	6–9%	
Stearic Acid	2.4–6%	
Alpha-Linolenic Acid	0.3–1%	
Palmitoleic Acid	0.5–0.7%	C16:1
Vitamin E	14 IU	

HAZELNUT OIL

Oleic Acid	65–85%
Linoleic Acid	7–11%

Palmitic Acid	4–6%	
Stearic Acid	2–4	
Unsaponifiables	0.3–1%	

HEMP SEED OIL

Linoleic Acid	53–60%	
Alpha-Linolenic Acid	15–25%	
Oleic Acid	8.5–16%	
Palmitic Acid	6–9%	
Stearic Acid	2–3.5%	
Gamma-Linolenic Acid	1–4%	C18:3
Arachidic Acid	1–3%	C20:0
Stearidonic Acid	0.4–2%	C18:4
Eicosanoic Acid	<.5%	C20:1
Behenic Acid	<.3%	C22:0

ILLIPE BUTTER

Stearic Acid	39–50%	
Oleic Acid	31–40%	
Palmitic Acid	10–23%	
Arachidic Acid	1–3%	C20:0
Linoleic Acid	1–2%	
Myristic Acid	1½%	C14:0
Unsaponifiables	0.5–1%	

JOJOBA OIL

Eicosenoic Acid	50–80%	C20:1
Docosenoic/Erucic Acid1	4–20%	C22:1
Oleic Acid	10–25%	
Palmitic Acid	<4%	

Palmitoleic Acid	<1%	C16:1
Stearic Acid	<1%	
Alpha-Linolenic Acid	<1%	

KARANJ OIL

Oleic Acid	45–72%	
Linoleic Acid	11–18%	
Eicosenoic Acid	9–12%	C20:1
Behenic Acid	4.2–5.3%	C22:0
Palmitic Acid	3.7–7.9%	
Arachidic Acid	2.2–4.7%	C20:0
Stearic Acid	2.4–8.9%	
Lignoceric Acid	1.1–3.5%%	C24:0

KIWI SEED OIL

Alpha-Linolenic Acid	45–70%	
Linoleic Acid	17–22%	
Oleic Acid	10½–14%	
Stearic Acid	4–7%	
Palmitic Acid	4–6%	
Arachidic Acid	0–1%	C20:0
Eicosenoic Acid	0–½%	C20:1

KOKUM BUTTER

Stearic Acid	50–62%	
Oleic Acid	30–42%	
Palmitic Acid	2–6%	C16:1
Linoleic Acid	0–2%	
Arachidic Acid	1.2%	C20:0

KUKUI NUT OIL

Linoleic Acid	35–50%	
Alpha-Linolenic Acid	25–40%	
Oleic Acid	10–35%	
Palmitic Acid	4–10%	
Stearic Acid	2–8%	
Arachidonic Acid	<1.5%	C20:4
Lauric Acid	<1.0%	C12:0
Myristic Acid	<1.0%	C14:0
Unsaponifiables	<1%	

MACADAMIA NUT OIL

Oleic Acid	54–63%	
Palmitoleic Acid	16–23%	C16:1
Palmitic Acid	7–10%	
Stearic Acid	2–6%	
Arachidic Acid	1½–3%	C20:0
Linoleic Acid	1–3%	
Eicosenoic Acid	1–3%	C20:1

MANGO BUTTER

Oleic Acid	34–56%	
Stearic Acid	26–57%	
Palmitic Acid	3–18%	
Linoleic Acid	1–13%	
Arachidic Acid	1½–3%	C20:0
Unsaponifiables	1–5%	

MARULA OIL

Oleic Acid	70–78

Palmitic Acid	9–12	
Stearic Acid	5–8	
Linoleic Acid	4–7	
Myristic Acid	<1.5	C14:0
Arachidic Acid	<1.0	C20:0
Alpha-Linolenic Acid	1–0.7%	
Erucic Acid	<0.5	C22:1

MEADOWFOAM OIL

Gadoleic Acid	61.5%	C20:1
Brassic Acid	17.9%	C22:2
Erucic Acid	12.7%	C22:1
Oleic Acid	3.2%	C18:1

MILK THISTLE OIL

Linoleic Acid	46–65%	
Oleic Acid	15–25%	
Palmitic Acid	7–12%	
Stearic Acid	5%	
Behenic Acid	1–1.5%	C22:0
Arahinovaya Acid	1.5–2%?	

MORINGA OIL

Oleic Acid	73%	
Behenic Acid	7–10%	C22:0
Palmitic Acid	7%	
Stearic Acid	5.1%	
Arachidic Acid	3.6%	C20:0
Eicosenoic/Gadoleic Acid	2.3%	C20:1
Palmitoleic Acid	1.1%	C16:1

| Lignoceric Acid | 1.0% | C24:0 |
| Myristic Acid | 0.1% | C14:0 |

NEEM OIL

Oleic Acid	40–60%	
Stearic Acid	14–22%	
Palmitic Acid	14–19%	
Linoleic Acid	8–20%	
Arachidic Acid	<3.5%	C20:0
Myristic Acid	<3%	C14:0
Lauric Acid	<1%	C12:0
Alpha-Linolenic Acid	<0.8%	

NIGELLA/BLACK CUMIN SEED OIL

Linoleic Acid	57.9%	
Oleic Acid	23.7%	
Palmitic Acid	13.7%	
Stearic Acid	2.6%	
Arachidic Acid	1.3%	C20:0
Myristic Acid	0.5%	C14:0
Alpha-Linolenic Acid	0.2%	

OAT SEED OIL

Oleic Acid	35–43%	
Linoleic Acid	35–43%	
Palmitic Acid	14–16%	
Stearic Acid	1–2 %	
Alpha-Linolenic Acid	1–1.5%	
Lauric Acid	0.39%	C12:0
Avenic Acid	0.2–0.6%	C18:1

Palmitoleic Acid	0.2%	C16:1
Myristic Acid	0.1–0.5%	C14:0
Icosanoic Acid	0.5–1%	C20:1
Icosanoic Acid	0.05–0.15%	C20:0

OLIVE OIL

Oleic Acid	63–81%	
Linoleic Acid	5–15%	
Palmitic Acid	7–14%	
Stearic Acid	3–5%	
Palmitoleic Acid	<3%	C16:1
Alpha-Linolenic Acid.	5%	
Arachidic Acid	<0.7%	C20:0
Unsaponifiables	0.5–1%	

PALM OIL

Palmitic Acid	43–45%	
Oleic Acid	38–41%	
Linoleic Acid	9–11%	
Stearic Acid	4–5%	
Myristic Acid	0.5–2%	C14:0
Arachidic Acid	<0.5	C20:0
Lauric Acid	<0.5%	C12:0
Unsaponifiables	0.5–1.2%	

PALM KERNEL OIL

Lauric Acid	48%	C12:0
Myristic Acid	15%	C14:0
Oleic Acid	15%	
Palmitic Acid	9%	

Capric Acid	3.4%	C10:0
Caprylic Acid	3.3%	C 8:0
Stearic Acid	2.5%	
Linoleic Acid	2.3%	

PAPAYA SEED OIL

Oleic Acid	71.6%	
Palmitic Acid	15.1%	
Linoleic Acid	7.7%	
Stearic Acid	2.6%	
Arachidic Acid	0.87%	C20:0
Alpha-Linolenic Acid	0.6%	
Myristic acid	0.16%	C14:0
Lauric acid	0.13%	
Behenic acid	0.02%	C22:0

PASSION FRUIT OIL

Linoleic Acid	77%
Oleic Acid	12%
Palmitic Acid	8%
Stearic Acid	2%
Alpha-Linolenic Acid	1.5%

PEACH KERNEL OIL

Oleic Acid	55–67%
Linoleic Acid	25–35%
Palmitic Acid	5–8%
Stearic Acid	3%
Alpha-Linolenic Acid	1%
Palmitoleic Acid	1%

Arachidic Acid	0.5%	C20:0

PECAN OIL

Oleic Acid	52%
Linoleic Acid	36.6%
Palmitic Acid	7.1%
Stearic Acid	2.2%
Alpha-Linolenic Acid	1.5%

PEANUT OIL

Oleic Acid	46.8%	
Linoleic Acid	33.4%	
Palmitic Acid	10%	
Behenic Acid	2.8%	C22:0
Stearic Acid	2%	
Arachidic Acid	1.4%	C20:0
Gadoleic Acid	1.3%	C20:1
Lignoceric Acid	0.9%	C24:0
Myristic Acid	0.1%	C14:0
Palmitoleic Acid	0.1%	C16:1

PEQUI SEED OIL

Oleic Acid5	0.2%	
Palmitic Acid	44.3%	
Stearic Acid	1.8%	
Palmitoleic Acid	1.3%	C16:1
Linoleic Acid	1.2%	
Alpha-Linolenic Acid	0.7%	
Myristic Acid	0.5%	C14:0

PERILLA SEED OIL

Alpha-Linolenic Acid	45–65%	
Linoleic Acid	10–20%	
Oleic Acid	10–25%	
Palmitic Acid	3–9%	
Stearic Acid	0–4%	
Palmitoleic Acid	<1%	C16:1

PISTACHIO NUT OIL

Oleic Acid	51–54%	
Linoleic Acid	31–35%	
Palmitic Acid	9–12%	
Palmitoleic Acid	1–2%	C16:1
Stearic Acid	1–2%	
Alpha-Linolenic Acid	<1%	

PLUM KERNEL OIL

Oleic Acid	60–80%	
Linoleic Acid	15–25%	
Palmitic Acid	4–9%	
Stearic Acid	0.7–2.6%	
Alpha-Linolenic Acid	<1%	
Palmitoleic Acid	<1%	C16:1
Gondoic Acid	0.2%	C20:1
Arachidic Acid	<0.3%	C20:0
Margaric Acid	0.1%	C17:0
Myristic Acid	<0.1%	C14:0
Behenic Acid	<0.1%	C22:0
Lignoceric Acid	<0.1%	C24:0
Heptadecenoic Acid	<0.1%	C17:1

POMEGRANATE SEED OIL

Punicic Acid	70–76 %	C18:3
Linoleic Acid	7%	
Oleic Acid	5.7%	
Palmitic Acid	2%	
Stearic Acid	1.3–2 %	
Gadoleic Acid	trace	C20:0

POPPY SEED OIL

Linoleic Acid	70.6%	
Oleic Acid	15.5%	
Palmitic Acid	19.4%	
Stearic Acid	2.3%	
Alpha-Linolenic Acid	0.06%	
Palmitoleic Acid	0.15%	C16:1
Arachidic Acid	0.11%	C20:0
Gadoleic Acid	0.07%	C20:1
Myristic Acid	0.05%	C14:0

PRACAXI OIL

Oleic Acid	55%	
Linoleic Acid	20%	
Behenic Acid	10–25%	C22:0
Lignoceric Acid	10–15%	C24:0
Palmitic Acid	5%	C16:0
Palmitoleic Acid	5%	C16:1
Stearic Acid	5%	
Gadoleic Acid	1.5%	C20:1
Erucic Acid	1%	C22:1
Arachidic Acid	1%	C20:0

Alpha-Linolenic Acid	0.5%	
Myristic Acid	0.43%	C14:0
Lauric Acid	0.12%	C12:0

PUMPKIN SEED OIL

Linoleic Acid	55.3%	
Oleic Acid	26.4%	
Palmitic Acid	12.9%	
Stearic Acid	4.8%	
Arachidic Acid	0.3%	C20:0

RED RASPBERRY OIL

Linoleic Acid	52.1%
Alpha-Linolenic Acid	22.2%
Oleic Acid	11.7%
Palmitic Acid	2%
Stearic Acid	0.9%

RICE BRAN OIL

Oleic Acid	32–38%
Linoleic Acid	32–47%
Palmitic Acid	13–23%
Stearic Acid	2–3%
Alpha-Linolenic Acid	1–3%
Unsaponifiables	3–4%

ROSEHIP SEED OIL

Linoleic Acid	43–46%
Alpha-Linolenic Acid	31–35%
Oleic Acid	15%

Palmitic Acid	3–4%	
Stearic Acid	1.5–2.5%	
Arachidic Acid	0.9%	C20:0
Myristic Acid	0.3%	C14:0
Eicosanoic Acid	0.5%	C20:0
Behenic	0.4%	C22:0
Unsaponifiables	0.8%	

SACHA INCHI OIL

Alpha-Linolenic Acid	45–51%
Linoleic Acid	32–37%
Oleic Acid	9–10.5%
Palmitic Acid	3–5%
Stearic Acid	2–4%

SAFFLOWER OIL—Hi-Linoleic

Linoleic Acid	70–80%	
Oleic Acid	10–20%	
Palmitic Acid	6–7%	
Stearic Acid	2.5–7%	
Alpha-Linolenic Acid	<0.5%	
Arachidic Acid	<0.5%	C20:0
Unsaponifiables	0.5–1.5%	

SAL BUTTER

Stearic Acid	41–47%	
Oleic Acid	37–43%	
Palmitic Acid	4–7%	
Arachidonic Acid	3–9%	C20:4
Linoleic Acid	0–4%	

Unsaponifiables	0.6–2.2%	

SEA BUCKTHORN SEED OIL

Linoleic Acid	34–35%	
Alpha-Linolenic Acid	32%	
Palmitic Acid	11%	
Oleic Acid	9%	
Elaidic Acid (a trans isomer of oleic acid)	5.6%	
Stearic Acid	4%	
Palmitoleic Acid	1.2%	C16:1

SEA BUCKTHORN FRUIT OIL

Palmitoleic Acid	34%	C16:1
Palmitic Acid	30.4	
Elaidic Acid (a trans isomer of oleic acid)	14.6	
Oleic Acid	7.1%	
Linoleic Acid	5.8%	
Alpha-Linolenic Acid	2.1%	
Myristic Acid	1.5%	C14:0

SESAME OIL

Oleic Acid	35–50%	
Linoleic Acid	35–50%	
Palmitic Acid	7–12%	
Stearic Acid	3.5–6%	
Alpha-Linolenictrace	–1%	
Eicosenoic Acidtrace	–1%	C20:0
Palmitoleic Acidtrace	–.5%	C16:1

SHEA BUTTER/SHEA STEARIN

Oleic Acid	40–55%
Stearic Acid	35–40%
Palmitic Acid	3–7%
Linoleic Acid	3–8%
Unsaponifiables	17%

SHEA OIL/SHEA OLEIN

Oleic Acid	73%
Linoleic Acid	14%
Stearic Acid	8.5%
Palmitic Acid	4%
Alpha-Linolenic Acid	0.35%

SHEA NILOTICA

Oleic Acid	40–55%	
Stearic Acid	30–32%	
Linoleic Acid	3–11%	
Palmitic Acid	4–9%	
Alpha-Linolenic Acid	<1%	
Arachidic Acid	<1%	C20:0

SOYBEAN OIL

Linoleic Acid	46–53%
Oleic Acid	22–27%
Palmitic Acid	10–12%
Alpha-Linolenic Acid	8–9%
Stearic Acid	5–6%
Unsaponifiables	0.5–1.6%

SUNFLOWER OIL

Linoleic Acid	72%	
Oleic Acid	15.9%	
Palmitic Acid	5.8%	
Stearic Acid	3.9%	
Behenic Acid	0.7%	C22:0
Alpha-Linolenic Acid	0.6%	
Tetracosanoic Acid	0.5%	C24:0
Arachidic Acid	0.3%	C20:0
Gadoleic Acid	0.2%	C20:1
Gamma-Linolenic Acid	0.1%	C18:3
Palmitoleic Acid	0.1%	C16:1

TOMATO SEED OIL

Linoleic Acid	50%	
Palmitic Acid	20–29%	
Oleic Acid	13–18%	
Stearic Acid	3%	
Alpha-Linolenic Acid	2–3%	
Arachidic Acid	<3%	C20:0
Behenic Acid	<1%	C22:0
Erucic Acid	<1%	C22:1

WALNUT OIL

Linoleic Acid	45–65%
Oleic Acid	25–35%
Alpha-Linolenic Acid	9–15%
Palmitic Acid	5–8%
Stearic Acid	3–73%

Unsaponifiables	½–1%

WATERMELON SEED OIL

Linoleic Acid	55–65%
Oleic Acid	21–29%
Palmitic Acid	8–13%
Stearic Acid	1.5–5.5%
Alpha-Linolenic Acid	<2%
Palmitoleic Acid<	1%

WHEAT GERM OIL

Linoleic Acid	55–60%
Oleic Acid	13–39%
Palmitic Acid	13–20%
Alpha-Linolenic Acid	4–10%
Stearic Acid	2–6%
Unsaponifiables	3–4%

YANGU OIL/CAPE CHESTNUT

Oleic Acid	45%	
Linoleic Acid	29%	
Palmitic Acid	18.3%	
Stearic Acid	4.7%	
Alpha-Linolenic Acid	0.9%	
Icosanoic Acid	0.5%	C20:0
Docosanoic/Erucic Acid	0.1%	C22:1

Measurements and Equivalents

8 oz	1 cup		240 ml		
4 oz	½ cup	8 tbs.	120 ml		
2 oz	⅓ cup	4 tbs	50 ml		
1 oz	1/8 cup	2 tbs.	30 ml	6 tsp.	
½ oz		1 tbs.	15 ml	3 tsp.	
			5 ml	1 tsp	100 drops
			2.5 ml	½ tsp	50 drops
				¼ tsp	25 drops

ESSENTIAL OIL DILUTIONS BY PERCENTAGE

Essential oils are strong plant compounds and should not be used undiluted on the skin. The following table lays out the relationship between drops and percentage dilutions for different volumes of oil. For example, in a one-ounce bottle of lavender massage oil you would add six drops of lavender essential oil for a 1% dilution. If combining more than one essential oil scent the total could add up to six drops, i.e., three drops lavender and three drops geranium

Percentage		1%	2%	2.50%	3%	4%	5%	10%
ML	Oz							
5 ml	1/6 oz	1	2	2.5	3	4	5	10
10 ml	1/3 oz	2	4	5	6	8	10	20
15 ml	1/2 oz	3	6	7.5	9	12	15	30
30 ml	1 oz	6	12	15	18	24	30	60
50 ml	<2oz	10	20	25	30	40	50	100
60ml	2 oz	12	24	30	36	28	60	120
100 ml		20	40	50	60	80	100	200
120ml	4 oz	24	48	60	72	96	120	240
240 ml	8oz	48	96	120	144	192	240	480
500ml	16oz	81	192	240	288	384	480	960

GLOSSARY OF
RELATED TERMS

Absolute: a solvent extraction of a plant, used when steam distillation would either harm the delicate aroma of the plant or flower or not result in an aromatic product.

Acid mantle: the natural, lightly acidic film on the surface of the skin produced by the sebaceous glands. As a viscous fluid, it helps protect the skin from bacteria, viruses, and other invasions.

Active principle: a term used to designate components of a product or recipe that are active agents in some aspect of the use of the product; i.e., sunscreen, emollient, humectant, therapeutic, nourishing, etc. Antonym: carrier principle.

Aerial parts: the above-ground parts of a plant or herb.

ALA: another common abbreviation for alpha-Linolenic acid, one of two essential fatty acids.

Alpha-Linolenic Acid (LNA): one of two essential fatty acids that need to be consumed in the diet.

Allergen: a substance that can cause a reaction in sensitive people but that is not an irritant or toxic to all people.

Analgesic: a term referring to pain-relieving properties.

Antibacterial: a substance that effectively kills bacteria.

Antioxidant: a substance that inhibits the oxidation process by reducing the number of free radical oxygen molecules that are released in biochemical reactions. They slow the formation of lipid peroxides and free radical oxygen forms, which damage cell membranes and other molecules. Examples include vitamin E, C, gum benzoin, rosemary extract, and carotenoids.

Aromatherapy: a term coined in 1928 in France by Rene-Maurice Gattefosse after he cured a serious burn on his arm using lavender essential oil. Aromatherapy involves applying the many aromatic compounds found in plants for therapeutic purposes.

Bacteriostatic: a substance that stops the growth of bacteria but does not kill it.

Barrier function: one of two functions of the stratum corneum, the protective function.

Base: in chemistry, this refers to substances that are low in H+ and high in OH- ions, and which fall between 7.5 and 14 pH.

Base: in soap- or cream-making, this can refer to the majority component in a product, or solubility, as in "oil-based" or "water-based."

Beta-carotene: the precursor of vitamin A from plant sources and an antioxidant carotenoid. It can also be used as a natural colorant.

Beta-sitosterol: a phytosterol (plant sterol) that has been shown to lower serum cholesterol levels. It is found in the unsaponifiable portion of oils and fats.

Botanical: indicates the source of a substance or image is from plants.

Buffer: something that mitigates the effects of a substance. For example, the acetic acid in vinegar can buffer the effect of spilt sodium hydroxide solution; weak acid buffering base.

Butter, vegetable: a saturated fat of vegetable origin, usually from the tropical regions; shea butter, mango butter, and sal butter are examples.

Carotenoids: phyto elements that play a major role in photo protection from sunlight in the cells and tissues. Carotenoids also play a large role as antioxidants in food and in the body. There are over 600 identified carotenoids and these include beta-carotene, lycopene, alpha carotene, lutein, canthaxanthin, and zeaxanthin.

Carrier principle: refers to a substance that carries another substance; as an example, a vegetable oil acting as a carrier for an essential oil, or the base carrier of active agents in a product. Antonym: active principle.

Ceramides: a mix of lipids and skin cells, corneocytes, that make up the outermost layer of skin, the stratum corneum.

Cinnamic acid: a polyphenolic natural plant-based sun protective agent found in shea butter and other oils.

Cold pressing:-Usually for fixed oils, and refers to the process of extracting the oils through the use of pressure rather than solvents. Only low amounts of heat should be generated by the process, thus "cold pressing."

Cold process soap-making: The oils and lye are mixed at relatively low temperatures of 80° to 110° F, and no additional heat is added to the process. The term is relative, comparing it to the more common hot process soaps in industry where the fat is boiled.

Collagen: One third of the body's connective tissue of the skin is made of collagen. The aging process takes place when the collagen becomes insoluble and incapable of absorbing moisture. When the skin is young the collagen is soluble, supple, and able to hold moisture.

Comedogenic: promotes acne and skin blockage. "Comedo" means a blackhead from a clogged sebaceous gland. *Comedo*, Latin, -glutton. Non-comedogenic, in cosmetics, means that the substance does not add a barrier layer on the skin that can clog pores.

Concrete: a solvent extraction of a plant to obtain an aromatic substance. Concretes need further treatment with alcohol to obtain an absolute.

Conjugated fatty acids: fatty acids that have both cis and trans configuration naturally, causing oils to be fuller feeling than the more normal cis configuration of fatty acids.

Corneocytes: dead skin cells that make up the ceramides of the stratum corneum, and that are bound together with the lipids of the sebum. Includes waxes, cholesterol, and free fatty acids.

Dermis: the middle layer of the three layers of skin, also called the cutis.

Dry oils: oils that contain tannins and have a *dry* feeling on the skin, not an oily feeling. These oils are high in tannins that create this dryness.

Drying oils: oils containing a significant percentage of poly and superunsaturated fatty acids, that dry to the touch by oxidation over time.

Elaidic acid: a trans isomer of oleic found naturally in very small amounts in cow and goat products and a major trans fat found in hydrogenated oils.

Emollience: describes substances that soften and soothe the skin, acting as a barrier against the environment by preventing moisture loss from the tissues.

Epidermis: the skin's outermost layer, consisting of five sub layers.

EPO: evening primrose oil

Essential Fatty Acids, EFAs: Fats that cannot be synthesized in the body but must be taken into the body in the form of food or transdermally, through the skin. There are two EFAs, linoleic and alpha-Linolenic acids. They have also been given a vitamin name, vitamin F, which is seldom used.

Essential nutrients: are necessary nutrients, catalysts, and cofactors that must be taken in by the body in foods. This includes the vitamins, eight amino acids, minerals, essential fatty acids, air, sunlight and water.

Essential oil: the "essence" of a plant, the natural oils that make up the scent and aroma properties of plants. These are short-chained, volatile, dispersing oils that come from plant parts; flowers, leaves, roots, needles, peels, bark, resins, seeds, and rhizomes.

Fatty acids (FAs): long chains of varying numbers of carbon atoms with hydrogen atoms connected to most or all of the carbon atoms. They consist of long hydrocarbon chains attached to carboxyl groups. Three fatty acids and a glycerol molecule make up a triglyceride.

Ferulic acid: a phyto, or plant, polyphenolic compound responsible for forming cell walls of plants, seed and bud break, as well as suppression and protection against microorganisms and pests in the plant. When used on the skin, it provides potent membrane antioxidant activity, suppresses melanin generation, prevents tanning, and absorbs and protects against ultraviolet wave damage. It is found in significant quantities in rice bran oil.

Fractionation: a process of separating triglycerides and fatty acids into their different physical properties. Using heat to liquefy oils, they are then cooled to a temperature between complete melting and solidification. The saturated molecules of the oil, which have a higher melting point, solidify and form crystals, while unsaturated fatty acids will remain in the liquid state. The crystalline part and the liquid part can be separated by filtration, and the oil is in effect divided into two *fractions*. This process is also done using chemicals and solvents.

Fragrance oil: a scented oil that could be totally synthetic or part synthetic and part essential oil. These oils were developed to provide inexpensive scenting properties to soaps, perfumes, household products, etc. They have no healing or therapeutic properties as essential oils do.

Free fatty acids: the fatty acids that are not bound to a glycerol molecule in the form of a triglyceride, but exist independently in a "free" state. Free fatty acids can cause instability in oil, causing it to go rancid sooner, as they are not chemically bound within the oil.

GLA, gamma-Linolenic acid: made from the essential fatty acid linoleic acid in the body and necessary for the production of prostaglandins, a hormone-like substance required for healthy functioning of the body. GLA was originally discovered in evening primrose oil, and has now been found to be particularly high in borage seed oil and black currant seed oils.

Glyceride: are esters formed by glycerol and fatty acids. Glycerol has three hydroxyl groups that can be combined with one, two, or three fatty acids to form monoglycerides, diglycerides, or triglycerides. Most oils and fats contain triglycerides which can be broken down by enzymes to form the mono and di forms of glycerides.

Glycerin: a by-product of soap making. In order to make soap from oils, triglycerides are exposed to an alkali to break the molecule into its three fatty acid and glycerol molecules. The glycerol becomes glycerin in the reaction to the hydroxide ions.

Glycerol: a component of triglycerides, with one glycerol molecule and three fatty acid molecules. During the soap-making process, following hydrolysis the glycerol separates from the fatty acids and becomes free glycerin. Two glycerol molecules can be linked together to make a sugar molecule.

GMO: short for Genetically Modified Organism. While the FDA added GMOs to the GRAS list (see below) in 1992, stating that they were "substantially equivalent" to conventional crops, no comprehensive studies that aren't associated with the industry have been published. As of 2014 there is substantial push-back against this decision.

Grapefruit Seed Extract: a preservative that can be added to soap or topical cream to prolong its shelf life.

GRAS, Generally Regarded As Safe: a designation by the FDA that labels foods and supplements with a history of traditional use as safe. When a material is given the designation, new regulations are not required before it is approved for use by the public. This was done for GMOs in 1992 (see above).

Humectants: substances that attract and hold water. They act as moisturizers for the skin. Example: glycerin.

Hydro: in composition, like, of, or by means of water.

Hydrogen: a gas (atomic number symbol, H) that in combination with oxygen (O) produces water, H2O.

Hydrolysis: the state of chemical decomposition or ionic dissociation, chemical break-up, caused by water. Hydrolyzed is the state of something that has been subjected to hydrolysis—chemical decomposition by water.

Hydrogenation: the process of making an unsaturated oil into a saturated fat by adding hydrogen atoms to the double bonds of unsaturated fatty acids. Shortening and margarine are examples.

Hydrophilic: the attraction of a molecule to water.

Hydrophobic: molecules that are repelled by water.

Hypodermis: the lowermost skin layer closest to the musculature of the body, also sometimes called the sub-dermis.

INCI, International Nomenclature Cosmetic Ingredients: a standard labeling system for cosmetics used worldwide.

IUPAC: International Union of Pure and Applied Chemistry. One of their tasks is to set systematic and recognized names for chemical compounds.

Infuse: to macerate or soak plant material in a substance such as vegetable oil, alcohol, or vinegar, to extract the therapeutic properties from the plant into the oil or other medium.

Iodine value: measures a fat or oil's saturation, i.e., the amount of iodine chloride the fat or oil can absorb. Saturated fats have low iodine values, while unsaturated oils have high numbers, depending on the degree of unsaturation.

Isomer: meaning "another name." A term used in chemistry for compounds that share the same chemical formula but have a different arrangement of atoms. They are not identical but are very similar.

IU, International Units: a unit of measure for use with some nutritional supplements, usually vitamin E and vitamin A.

LA: linoleic acid, one of two essential fatty acids.

LNA: alpha-Linolenic acid, one of two essential fatty acids.

Linoleic Acid (LA): one of two *essential* fatty acids that need to be consumed in the diet.

Lipids: the saponifiable portion of fats, oils, or waxes, the fatty acids and triglycerides. They are primarily hydrocarbon-like and insoluble in water.

Lipo: pertaining to fats, lipids. *Lipos* is the Greek word for fat.

Lipophilic: oil-loving or attracting, used to describe properties of molecules.

Lipophobic: oil-repelling, used to describe properties of molecules.

Long-chained fatty acids: carbon chain lengths from fourteen to eighteen carbon atoms.

Medium-chained fatty acids: fatty acid chains with carbon lengths from eight to twelve carbon atoms.

Melanin: the cellular pigment structure in the skin that dissipates the effect of the sun by darkening the skin, making it less susceptible to damage from UVB rays.

Melting point: the melting point of an oil is determined by its fatty acid chain lengths and saturation.

Metabolites: intermediate compounds that form a bridge between raw materials in food and their destination in the body processes.

Mineral oil: made from petroleum products. Often found in cosmetics and baby oil, it is not considered a "natural" product for healthy skin.

Miscibility: the ability to dissolve in, become one with another substance, as molasses dissolves in water.

Monounsaturated: oils that have only one carbon-to-carbon double bond in the fatty acid chain.

MUFA: monounsaturated fatty acid.

Mucilage: a slimy, slippery substance from plants, which can protect the mucus membranes of the body. They are mild and play a part in the treatment of gastritis and other stomach disorders.

Nitrilosides: vitamin B-17, from apricot kernels and other plant seeds. They are a part of laetrile cancer therapy.

Non-polar: in chemistry, a substance that resists water. Waxes are extremely non-polar.

Occlusive, Occlude: to shut out or in. An occlusive film is a layer of oil protecting the skin below, or blocking natural respiratory process.

Oil: a term for lipids and non-lipid compounds produced by seeds and nuts of the plant world, and which also includes animal and petrochemical oils.

Omega designation of fatty acids: determined by the number of carbon atoms from the free fatty end to the first double bond in an unsaturated fatty acid.

Organic: a growing method that uses natural growing practices to emphasize the health of a plant or crop rather than relying on synthetic fertilizers and pesticides.

—pertaining to, derived from, of the nature of an organ, life.

—chemistry, concerned with carbon compounds. Carbon compounds are found in things that were once alive.

Oxidation: a process similar to combustion that happens in the presence of oxygen in biochemical reactions. In the body, free radical oxygen molecules cause damage at the cellular level.

Passage function: the secondary function of the stratum corneum, the function of movement of substances in and out of the outer skin layer. Barrier function is the primary function of the stratum corneum.

Percutaneous: made from two words, beyond, *peri-*, and skin, *cutis*, meaning absorbed into and beyond the skin into the body.

Phenolic compounds: a class of chemical compounds produced by plants and microorganisms. It consists of a hydroxyl group bonded to an aromatic hydrocarbon group. Organisms produce phenolic compounds in response to environmental conditions, insects, UV radiation, and damage to tissues. Polyphenols means multiple phenols. Phenolic compounds can also be industrially synthesized.

Phospholipids: lipid compounds found in living cells of animals and plants, which are important for healthy skin and body cells. Lecithin is a well-known phospholipid.

Physiologic: from *physi(o)* Greek for nature and *logos*, discourse, the study of the life of nature, plants, and animals. Used to describe something in keeping with the maintenance of health in plants or animals.

Phyto: the Latin word for plant.

Phytosterols: the vegetable analogues of cholesterol. They are essential cell membrane components and necessary for an efficient immune system. Beta-sitosterol, sitosterol, campesterol, stigmasterol, and sitostanol are examples of some phytosterols.

Polar: a term in chemistry that means a substance can dissolve in water, attracts water.

PL: phospholipids.

Polyunsaturated: oils that have at least two carbon-to-carbon double bonds in their fatty acid chain.

Preservative: something that preserves something else from deterioration. There are different actions performed by preservatives. Antioxidants preserve oils by preventing the deterioration of the oils from the oxidation process, while bactericides and fungicides kill or retard the growth of bacterial and other molds and conditions that will spoil a product.

SAP value: the amount of KOH, potassium hydroxide, necessary to turn oil into soap.

Saponification: the chemical action that occurs when making soap from oil and alkali. It can also be viewed as the breaking down of the ingredients into parts, and the reaction of those parts with each other to form soap.

Saponins: formed in plants, these are a group of plant glycosides in which water-soluble sugars are attached to a lipophilic steroid or triterpenoid, resulting in a hydrophobic/hydrophilic asymmetry that lowers surface tension and is soap-like.

SaFA: saturated fatty acids

Saturated fatty acid: refers to the fact that all the carbon atoms of the fatty acid chain are *saturated* with hydrogen atoms. This includes fats and oils that are generally solid at room temperature, and applies to all animal fats and some vegetable fats. Lauric, myristic, palmitic, and stearic acids are saturated.

Sebaceous glands: glands in the skin that are attached to hair follicles and produce a fine protective film of lipids to protect the skin. The "acid mantle" is another name for this film.

Sebum: the fatty, or lipid, product of the skin that is produced by the sebaceous glands. Sebum serves to lubricate and protect the skin from the environment, preventing evaporation of moisture by holding moisture in the skin layer.

Short-chained fatty acids: fatty acids with carbon chain lengths of up to six carbon atoms.

Soap: the product that results when a slightly acidic fatty acid and a strong base react, producing a slightly basic salt called soap. Also, the salt of a fatty acid and a metal. For most, soap is used to wash with. However there are other chemical processes that produce soap that would be unrecognizable to most of us.

Sperm whale oil: a type of highly desired oil produced from sperm whales in the eighteenth, nineteenth, and early twentieth centuries. Jojoba oil and meadowfoam seed oils were developed in the 1970s as farmed alternatives.

Squalene: a natural part of our skin sebum or lipids, produced by the sebaceous glands in the epidermis. Vegetable sources of squalene are found in olive oil, wheat germ oil, and rice bran oils. Animal sources include shark liver oil.

Stratum corneum: the outermost layer of the five layers of the epidermis. Meaning "horned layer" in Latin, it was once thought to be an inert film but is now considered biologically active.

Stearic acid: a fatty acid occurring naturally in tallow and other animal fats and vegetable oils. *Stea-* is the root of the Greek word for fat. It is often used in soap and cosmetics for its smoothness and hardness, but is a sensitizer for some allergic people.

Sterols: natural compounds found in plants and animals, which have many vital biological functions. Cholesterol and beta-sitosterol are well-known sterols. Hormones such as testosterone, estrogen, progesterone, and corticosteroids are made from cholesterol in the body and are considered modified sterols.

Stigmasterol: the phytosterol known as the anti-stiffness factor, found in significant quantities in shea butter's unsaponifiable portion. In Africa, shea butter is used to massage arthritic joints and sore muscles.

Super unsaturated: oils that have three or more carbon to carbon double bonds in the fatty acid chain.

Surfactant: surface active agent; surf-ac-tant. A substance that will unite oil and water, so that the molecular bonds of water are broken and spread smoothly over a surface, rather than beading up. Soap is an example.

Tallow: the fat from animals; including cattle, sheep, and horses. Lard is the fat of pigs.

Terpenes: a class of hydrocarbons widely occurring in plants and animals. Made up of recurring isoprene units (5 hydrocarbons, C5H8), they are vital to the functioning and structure of living organisms.

Terpenoid: a similar structure to the terpenes, with the addition of oxygen atoms.

TEWL, Trans Epidermal Water Loss: a designation used in the cosmetic industry to indicate the moisture retentive properties of the skin when using various substances.

TG: triglycerides

Tocopherol: is one form of vitamin E, and a preservative against oxidation. Produced by most plants for protection, it is part of the unsaponifiable portion of fats and oils and helps to keep them from oxidizing.

Tocotrienols: a class of the vitamin E group. Smaller and less saturated than the tocopherols, they are potent antioxidants. Some plants produce them in their oils, but not all.

Tocomonoenol: a recently discovered branch of the vitamin E group, and another antioxidant, found in kiwi seed and peel.

Topical: refers to the application of oils, creams, or other substances applied to the skin. External treatment.

Trans-fatty acids: a type of industrially produced fatty acid formed when polyunsaturated acids are made saturated or partially saturated. They have been found to harm our health.

Triglycerides: three fatty acid molecules and one glycerol molecule.

Unsaponifiables: the parts of the oils and fats that cannot be decomposed into an acid, an alcohol or a salt (soap). In other words, the part of oil not made into soap during the soap-making process. Carrying nourishing elements such as proteins, vitamins, and sterols, they remain in soaps, but are not turned into soap molecules.

Unsaturated fatty acids: those where carbon chains are missing hydrogen atoms in several places. These are oils that are liquid at room temperature and usually derived from vegetable sources. Oleic, linoleic, palmitoleic, gamma-Linolenic acid are some of the unsaturated fatty acids.

Vegetable butter: saturated plant oils produced in or near the tropics that are solid at room temperature.

Very-long-chained fatty acids: those with carbon chain lengths of twenty carbon atoms and above.

Vitamin A: a necessary vitamin that is initiated by provitamin A compounds in foods and plants. Carotenoids act as provitamin A compounds, transforming to vitamin A in the body. Helpful for skin conditions such as acne.

Vitamin C: a necessary nutrient for the health of the skin and body. One of the essential nutrients, vitamin C protects cell walls, supports collagen health, and aids in skin repair.

Vitamin E: a family of related phenolic compounds that act as antioxidants and serve to protect cells. Added to oils to prolong their shelf life. Grouped in three branches, they are tocopherols, tocotrienols, and tocomonoenols.

Vitamin F: an outdated term for the two essential fatty acids, linoleic and alpha-Linolenic acids.

Vitamin P: an older term for the flavonoids.

Volatile: a dispersing, expanding substance. Essential oils are volatile, as they will completely evaporate into the atmosphere.

Wax: a class of lipids that are non-polar and do not contain a glycerol compound.

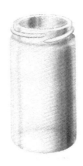

BIBLIOGRAPHY

BOOKS REFERENCED IN THE TEXT

Erasmus, Udo, *Fats that Heal, Fats that Kill*, Alive Books, Burnaby, BC, Canada, 1993.

Fife, Bruce, *Coconut Cures*, Piccadilly Books Ltd., Colorado Springs, CO, 2005.

Naiman, Ingrid, *Cancer Salves, A Botanical Approach to Treatment*, North Atlantic Books, Berkeley, CA, 1999.

Pelikan, Wilhelm, *Healing Plants, Insights Through Spiritual Science*, Mercury Press, Spring Valley, NY, 1997.

OTHER RESOURCES

Aromatherapy

Davis, Patricia, *Aromatherapy, An A–Z*, C.W. Daniel Company, Saffron Walden, England, 1995.

Keville, Kathi and Mindy Green, *Aromatherapy: A Complete Guide to the Healing Art*, The Crossing Press, Freedom, CA, 1995.

Lavabre, Marcel, *Aromatherapy Workbook*, Healing Arts Press, Rochester, VT, 1990.

Rose, Jeanne, *The Aromatherapy Book*, North Atlantic Books, Berkeley, CA, 1992.

Sellar, Wanda, *The Directory of Essential Oils*, C.W. Daniel Company, Saffron Walden, England, 1992.

Schnaubelt, Kurt, *Medical Aromatherapy*, Frog Ltd. Books, Berkeley, CA, 1999.

Schnaubelt, Kurt, *Advanced Aromatherapy*, trans. from German by J. Michael Beasley, Healing Arts Press, Rochester, VT, 1995.

Tisserand, Robert B., *The Art of Aromatherapy*, Healing Arts Press, Rochester, VT, 1977.

Tisserand, Robert B., *Aromatherapy, To Heal and Tend the Body*, Lotus Press, Wilmot, WI, 1988.

Natural Cosmetics & Skin Care

Cousin, Pierre Jean, *Facelift at Your Fingertips*, Storey Publishing, Pownal, VT, 2000.

Anti-Wrinkle Treatments for Perfect Skin, Storey Publishing, Pownal, VT, 2001.

Kellar, Casey, *The Natural Beauty and Bath Book*, Lark Books, Asheville, NC, 1997.

Hampton, Aubrey, *Natural Organic Hair and Skin Care*, Organica Press, Tampa, Florida, 1987.

What's in Your Cosmetics?, Odonian Press, Tuscon, AZ, 1995.

Hayes, Alan, *Health Scents*, Angus and Robertson/Harper Collins Publishers, Pymble, Sydney, NSW, Australia, 1995.

Rose, Jeanne, *Jeanne Rose's Herbal Body Book*, Perigee Books, The Berkeley Publishing Group, NY, 1976.

Smeh, Nikolaus J., *Health Risks in Today's Cosmetics*, Alliance Publishing Co., Garrisonville, VA, 1994.

Creating Your Own Cosmetics, Alliance Publishing Co.,
Garrisonville, VA, 1995.

Herbal Books

Gladstar, Rosemary, *Herbal Healing for Women*, Simon & Schuster, New
York, 1993.

Weed, Susun, *Healing Wise*, Ash Tree Pub., Woodstock, New York, 1989.

Breast Cancer? Breast Health!, Ash Tree Pub., Woodstock, New
York, 1996.

(Note: Other books by these two authors are also recommended.)

Edwards, Gail Faith, *Opening Our Wild Hearts to the Healing Herbs*, Ash
Tree Pub., Woodstock, New York, 2000.

Soap-Making Books

Cavitch, Susan Miller, *The Natural Soap Book*, Storey Publishing, Pownal,
VT, 1995.

Cavitch, Susan Miller, *The Soapmaker's Companion*, Storey Publishing,
Pownal, VT, 1997.

Cross, Melinda, *The Handmade Soap Book*, Storey Publishing, Pownal, VT,
1998.

Failor, Catherine, *Transparent Soapmaking*, Rose City Press, Portland, OR,
1997.

Making Natural Liquid Soaps, Storey Publishing, Pownal, VT, 2000.

Kellar, Casey, *The Natural Beauty and Bath Book*, Lark Books, Asheville,
NC, 1997.

Makela, Casey, *Milk-Based Soaps*, Storey Publishing, Pownal, VT, 1997.

Mohr, Merilyn, *The Art of Soap Making*, Camden House Publishing,
Camden East, Ontario, 1979.

Parker, Susan M., *Making Soap; A Primary on Natural Soap Making*, published by the author, Sebastopol, CA, 2000.

White, Elaine C., *Soap Recipes*, Valley Hills Press, Starkville, MS, 1995.

WEBSITES

Barclay-Nichols, Susan, *Point of Interest!* (blog),
 http://swiftcraftymonkey.blogspot.com/

Natural Sourcing,
 http://www.naturalsourcing.com

"Secondary Metabolites," Weizmann Institute of Science,
 **http://www.weizmann.ac.il/plants/aharoni/
 PlantMetabolomeCourse/March142007.pdf**

The Campain Against Trans Fats in Food,
 http://www.tfx.org.uk/page0.html

"Skin Aging," Life Extension Foundation,
 https://www.lef.org/protocols/skin_nails_hair/skin_aging_01.htm

"The Plant Phenolic Compounds," Weizmann Institute of Science,
 **http://www.weizmann.ac.il/plants/aharoni/
 PlantMetabolomeCourse/May092007.pdf**

Dr. Mercola (an internet source on many areas of natural health, including healthful oils and fats as well as the necessity of vitamin D)
 http://www.mercola.com

MAGAZINES AND NEWSPAPERS

Oomaha, B. Dave et al., "Characteristics of raspberry (Rubus idaeus L.) seed oil," *Food Chemistry* 69 (2000), 187–193.

Teicholz, Nina, "The Questionable Link between Saturated Fat and Heart Disease," *Wall Street Journal*, May 6, 2014.

Walsh, Bryan, "Don't Blame Fat," *Time Magazine*, June 23, 2014.

Willett, Walter, "The Case for Banning Trans Fats," *Scientific American*, March 2014.

OTHER BOOKS

Rudin, Donald, *Omega-3 Oils, A Practical Guide*, Avery Publishing Group, Garden City, NY, 1996.

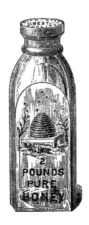

SOURCES

The internet is a vast resource that is accessible from any computer or laptop. The following are some of my favorite suppliers and comments about why I use them.

Mountain Rose Herbs

https://www.mountainroseherbs.com
PO Box 50220, Eugene, OR 97405
USA Toll-Free – (800) 879-3337, Outside USA – (541) 741-7307

Mountain Rose Herbs has many organic products and there is no minimum order or size limit.

Liberty Natural Products

http://www.libertynatural.com/index.html
20949 S. Harris Road, Oregon City, OR 97045
(800) 289-8427, or (503) 631-4488.

Liberty Natural is a wholesale supplier and has a $50 minimum.

Essential Wholesale

http://www.essentialwholesale.com,
2211 NW Nicolai St., Portland, OR 97210
(866) 252-9639

Essential Wholesale carries some organics and does not have a minimum purchase.

J. Edwards International

http://www.bulknaturaloils.com
141 Campanelli Dr., Braintree, MA 02184
(617) 472-9300

J. Edwards International has an excellent range of oils, many organic. The minimum size for most are 1 gallon, with a few others at 16 oz.

Soaper's Choice, a division of Columbus Foods

http://www.soaperschoice.com
30 E Oakton St., Des Plaines, IL 60018
(800) 322-6457 ext: 8930 or (847) 257-8930

Soaper's Choice also has a great range of oils, some organic, with a minimum size of 1 gallon.

From Nature With Love, a division of Natural Sourcing, LLC

http://www.fromnaturewithlove.com
341 Christian Street, Oxford, CT 0647
(800) 520-2060 or (203) 702-2500

Majestic Mountain Sage

https://www.thesage.com
2490 S 1350 W, Nibley, UT 84321
(435) 755-0863

Majestic Mountain Sage has a wide range of oils and other ingredients as well as a great soap calculator. No minimums and small sizes.

Organic Creations

http://www.organic-creations.com
2420 NW Campus Drive Suite E, Estacada, OR 97023
(503) 343-4992

A very wide range of raw materials.

Lotion Crafter

http://www.lotioncrafter.com
48 Hope Lane, Eastsound, WA 98245
(360) 376-8008

A wide variety of cosmetic raw materials, a few nice oils and incredibly fast shipping.

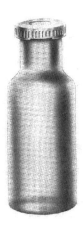

SOURCES FOR JARS, BOTTLES, AND OTHER SUPPLIES

Sunburst Bottles: http://www.sunburstbottle.com

A good source for small quantities of jars and bottles. They often have interesting shapes and colors of containers.

Specialty Bottle: http://www.specialtybottle.com

Another source for smaller quantities of jars and bottles.

SKS Bottle & Packaging: http://www.sks-bottle.com

518-880-6980, ext.1
An East Coast supplier of bottles and jars.

Salt Works: http://www.saltworks.us

An amazing number of different salts, including powdered, which makes for a lovely salt scrub.

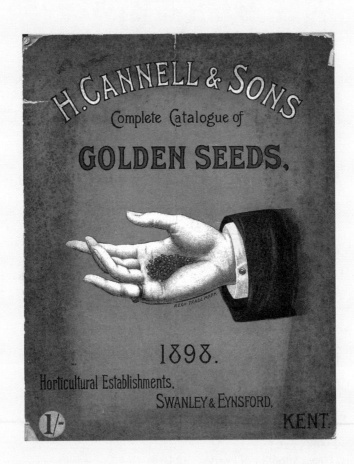

H. CANNELL & SONS

Complete Catalogue of

GOLDEN SEEDS,

REGᴰ TRADE MARK

1898.

Horticultural Establishments,

SWANLEY & EYNSFORD,

1/-

KENT.